How to use
Leg Wraps, Bandages and Boots

Supportive Leg Care for Your Horse

Written and illustrated by

Sue A. Allen

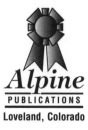

Alpine
PUBLICATIONS
Loveland, Colorado

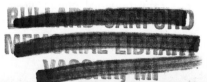

HOW TO USE LEG WRAPS, BANDAGES, AND BOOTS:
Supportive Leg Care for Your Horse

Copyright 1995 by Sue A. Allen

ISBN No. 0-931866-72-3

Library of Congress Cataloging in Publication information is available upon request.

Credits:

Edited by Dianne Borneman and B. J. McKinney.

Cover design and text layout by B J. McKinney.

Cover photos by Sue A. Allen.

This book is available at special quantity discounts for organizations, club promotions, premiums, or educational use. Write the publisher for details.

1 2 3 4 5 6 7 8 9 0

Printed in the United States of America.

In fond memory of Sen-sen

Acknowledgments

My gratitude goes to Richard C. Spike, DVM, of Swartz Creek, Michigan, who offered his expertise during the completion of this book. Dr. Spike, a graduate of Michigan State University, is also a licensed trainer and driver. He has covered Michigan-area-pony club shows and 4H exhibitions and has raced his Standardbreds during the seasons. Aiken, South Carolina will be claiming him part-time as one of its own by the time this book goes to press.

Appreciation also goes to the owners and handlers who gave their time and permission for photographing their horses at the Rhine Valley Farm, Rhinebeck, New York, Roseview Stables (HITS SHOWS), Poughkeepsie, New York, and The Millbrook Equestrian Center, Millbrook, New York. Farriers E. Dolan and M. Clina of the Hudson Valley, New York, were generous with information and advice. I express my heartfelt thanks to the students and the many others for assisting with the photography, to Jean Barbere and Sharon Miller for their help with illustrating the leg wraps, and to Dr. John Jagar for allowing photos of his veterinary examination. Many thanks to Weiss and Hawthorne Inc, of Dunkirk, Indiana, who supplied product information and illustrations; and to Herb and his employees at Lightning-G Tack, LaGrangeville, New York.

Many thanks to the contributors of photos and test results: Ulster International Inc., New Paltz, New York; Professionals Choice, Spring Valley, California; and Sporthorse Equipment, Petaluma, California.

Table of Contents

Introduction

This book is directed to individuals who want to learn how to maintain the best leg care possible for their horse. The legs of a performance horse are subject to continual stress and the potential for injury is high. Even the biggest boned, strongest Percheron has considerable sensitivity and requires as much care as the small-boned, delicate-appearing Arabian.

Preventive Maintenance

Preventive maintenance is stressed throughout this book, however, to achieve your goal of maintaining a sound and healthy horse, you must start with a good foundation, which means that you buy a healthy, sane horse with good structural conformation.

Good conformation starts with a horse's sire and dam. Many of the causes for a horse's leg and foot problems stem from faulty conformation or being too high strung, and such individual horses should never be asked to do more than they are capable of performing because of these flaws. Poor conformation in your horse's legs will be a plague if you are desirous of having a riding, driving, or racing horse. If you are about to purchase your first horse, it is advisable to hire a professional who is knowledgeable, such as a good horse trainer or riding instructor, or perhaps if you are taking riding lessons, someone who is expert from your riding school. Determining a sound horse with good leg conformation is

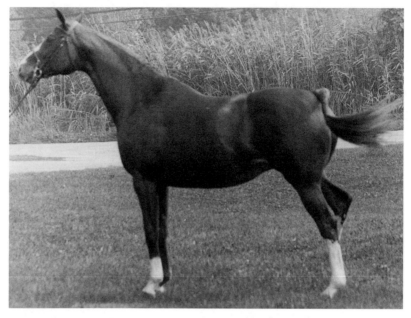

An excellent example of great conformation. This Thorougbred mare is posed in a stretch to show off her beauty.

for experts.

The purchase of your horse is certainly an important event, both financially as well as an entrance into a different lifestyle. A performance horse is an investment. He will be constantly dependent upon you for proper care and maintenance from the moment he is signed over to you. Many horse lovers compare a new horse in the barn to bringing home a new baby.

Investigate the way the seller maintains his horses. Your investment becomes less chancy when the horse has been well-maintained from foaling. Check the horse's barn records, if any, and ask questions about what kind of handling and/or riding has been done.

Correct maintenance and handling starts from the time the foal hits the ground. Care of his feet, environment, and handling with respect to good management is covered in the first chapter. Compare your potential horse's background to the simple routines and suggestions provided for you.

A second look a day or two later, if you are seriously interested in the horse, is generally wise. This is the occasion to take the professional you have hired along for an expert opinion. Your trainer will check the horse's way of going and look for physical qualities or defects. This close scrutiny is to reveal whether or not this horse suits your individual needs and abilities. If the horse meets all requirements and passes inspection, the next step is the vet check.

A medical pre-purchase examination is expensive, but you should consider it as an investment and part of the purchase price of the horse. It is also an occasion when you can become more familiar with your soon-to-be new horse's physical at-

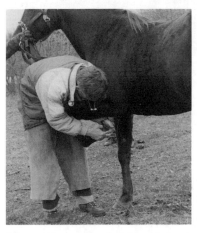

The vet flexes, then holds each front foot for about sixty seconds, then watches her being trotted out and back. The mare's first few strides will reveal her soundness.

Right: the rear is examined the same way for lameness or soreness in the rear leg joints and the quarters.

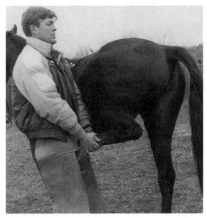

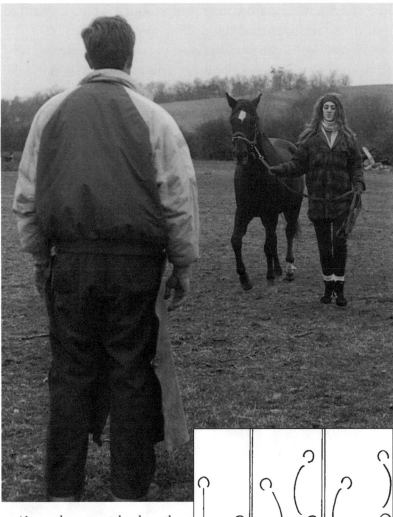

Above: the vet watches how the horse moves after each flexion.

Right: the travel line of all four feet. The first prints show the horse traveling in a fairly straight line. In the center set, the toes turn out, padding. This will cause interfering. On the right, the toe turns inward, with outward winging.

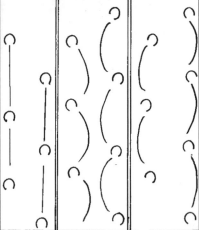

tributes and conformation. Most veterinarians will discuss each and every detail with the prospective buyer. That's what you're paying him for, isn't it?

A horse that is already being ridden or driven should have a soundness check. Often hidden soreness, which in an older horse is not unusual, is uncovered during this examination. The veterinarian can determine the seriousness of the condition. Most people do not want to purchase a great deal of vet bills along with the cost of the horse.

If you want a horse that is to jump and/or hunt, radiographing the joints of his lower legs is sometimes advised, particularly if showing is planned. After the horse passes all of these criteria, blood is drawn for a Coggins test. This is a prerequisite before purchase to assure the buyer he is not getting a horse infected with incurable equine infectious anemia. Several days may pass before the results of his Coggins and other tests are complete, which will give you some additional decision-making time. A vet who specializes in horses will point out any conformational faults also. Often it is not until a pre-purchase vet check that some fault or health problem comes to light. When you have reached this point in the sale, a negative finding can be very depressing; however, it is better to make this discovery before you make the purchase.

Buying a very young, unbroke horse is for only experienced horse people to undertake. Obtaining an unbroke horse that will remain sound well into its training depends on how he is put together, as well as how his sire and dam perform. Many specialized trainers who show prefer to buy a two-year-old horse because they want to start him out in a particular way of training and safeguard his legs.

Purchasing a horse or pony with fine overall conformation and a sane mind is a good start for a new owner. However, do not depend upon good conformation and a fine bill of health and soundness to guarantee a problem-free lifetime with any horse. Proper and consistent care of your horse is extremely important to assure good health and well being.

A horse's legs support his mobility. One leg at each "corner" holds him up and balances his weight. If one leg hurts, that corner collapses. When a horse becomes sore or injured, he is considered unsound until the injury heals and he is able to work again. The ideal situation is to always have a sound horse. So, it makes sense to do everything possible to protect his legs, helping them to remain sound and strong.

Leg Protection

A good maintenance program includes leg protection and support when needed. Bandaging a horse's lower legs is a conscientious way to safeguard them during training, schooling, and heavy workouts. Using leg bandages or correct boots can deter many injuries and avoid physical stress. If your horse is overworked or has a serious conformational fault, however, nothing can promise soundness.

Leg bandages and wraps are ordinarily made of cotton. They function as leg support and cushioning from the "ouches" while the horse is in motion or when he's tired or sore at the end of the day. Standing bandages and wraps are more than just a night-time comfort. They are also utilized when the horse has injured a leg or foot, as well as for therapeutic reasons.

The most commonly used leg wraps for working your horse are polo bandages. Polo bandages are made of cotton flannel and therefore wrap securely and will not slip or readily bind on your horse's legs during application, and they offer good support. If you are a beginner, I suggest that you start with polos. Once you know how to wrap with simple polos, it will be easier to use quilts and other kinds of wraps.

This book should help you understand the exact use of leg wraps and how to apply them correctly, as well as the various types of boots and their functions.

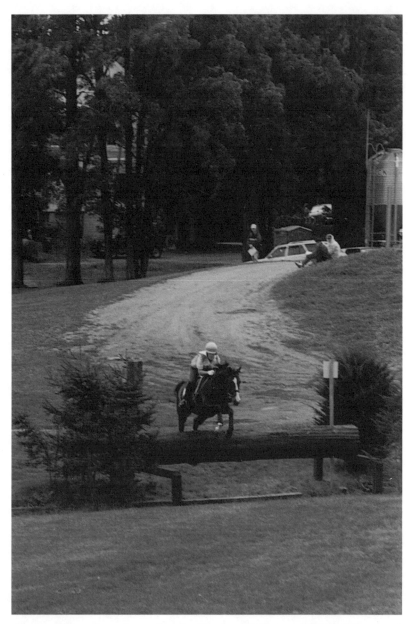

Clearing huge obstacles and galloping downhill on a field jumping run is extremely stressful on a horse's legs. Therefore, complete protection is utilized with brush boots or combination tendon/splint boots, plus bell boots.

CHAPTER 1
Keeping Your Horse's Legs Sound

Keeping your horse's legs and feet in prime working condition requires preventive maintenance. While wrapping or bandaging legs is the primary method of preventive maintenance covered in this book, it is important to pay attention to other routines that will help your horse have good legs and feet.

PREVENTIVE MAINTENANCE

For overall leg and foot care, you must follow these important guidelines:

Avoid training a young horse too soon, before his legs are solid enough. Working a young horse too soon can cause permanent damage to the legs. As the horse approaches his full growth, you can start ground driving or long-lining. Horses that will be driven are usually hitched shortly thereafter, at about twenty-six or twenty-eight months of age. Longeing in a circle less than sixty-five feet across or backing should not be done until the colt or filly is about three years of age. The growth and firmness of the front legs should be the deciding factors. Serious training should wait until the knee plates become strong enough to take tight turns and circles and hold a rider's weight. Splint boots and/or leg bandages will help protect these tender legs from stress.

A foal's feet must not be overlooked. His first trimming and foot evaluation should take place within his first month. Teach the foal to lead and allow his feet to be handled as early as possible. Your first concern is gaining his confidence and teaching him manners. Use short, patient training sessions and proceed at each individual foal's pace because his young body needs to build solid leg bones and muscle before much work can commence.

Avoid asking too much of an older horse that is out of condition. Older horses making a comeback (horses that have not worked for a year or so) should never be asked to do more than physically able either. Wrap the older horse's legs and work him about twenty minutes at walk and trot exercises. You may want to longe your horse a few times before saddling him if he has not been worked for several months. Wait until your horse begins to breathe easily and feels balanced to canter. Barrel racing, running, or jumping should be approached gradually to give your horse time to regain adequate strength and muscle. Overwork or physical stress during a comeback is a frequent cause of leg problems.

Establish Routine Hoof Care. Establish a routine of daily hoof cleaning and regular farrier visits. Daily, pick the dirt and debris from all four feet and check to make sure that no hoof damage has occurred since the last cleaning. When the feet are not cleaned every day, the soles become subject to injury and disease. A stone caught in the shoe or trapped in dirt on the bottom of a hoof can cause soreness. Muddy, wet feet and legs incubate bacteria. Fungus can colonize on the skin of pasterns and legs, while thrush may infest the cracks around the frogs of the feet under caked dirt and manure. Thrush thrives in dirty stall bedding or a damp barn. Dried-on mud dries out the hooves. Avoid these problems by washing the mud from legs and feet when you bring your horse in, and by cleaning his feet every day.

Find a Competent Farrier. Good farrier care is important whether the horse is shod or barefoot. Too many weeks between trimming and/or re-shoeing is an invitation to trouble. Damage to the feet, legs, and even the vertebrae can occur if shoes are left on too long. The hooves outgrow the shoes or the shoes are thrown off, hopefully witout tearing the hoof wall. Excessively long toes cause interference and stress within the legs. The unshod horse that is ridden almost daily will wear away much of his heels while the toes grow out, changing the angles of the foot. Regular trimming is necessary to maintain proper balance and prevent cracks in the hooves.

A quality farrier is the only farrier to permit near your horses. Good farriers are not miracle workers, but often it seems as if they are. These individuals are experts because of training and skills acquired in the trade while keeping abreast of current shoeing methods and foot appliances. Workshops and seminars help them improve their techniques.

A good farrier knows how to trim a horse's feet so each will land correctly and comfortably, and he takes pride in his work. When difficult problems arise, a foot specialist who is educated in therapeutic and specialized shoeing is able to work with your veterinarian if required.

Beware of inexperienced farriers who may not have apprenticed with an expert. If your horse's heels are trimmed off or other faulty trimming is done, whether arbitrarily or carelessly, the sudden change in the pastern angle could traumatize and stress your horse's legs. If correct balance is not restored immediately, your horse may become chronically lame.

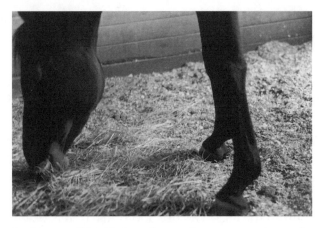

A clean, well-bedded stall contributes not only to the horse's comfort, but also to his good health.

Provide Good Care for Your Horse. Practice regular feeding and turnout programs in a safe environment. Horses that are content are less likely to injure themselves.

Balanced Diet. The nutritional balance in your horse's diet is important. Amino acids are essential for healthy hooves and coat. Grasses, such as meadow and orchard, should supply enough biotin and methionine, but when grazing is not possible or good timothy and grass hay is unavailable, these nutrients should be supplied in food supplements.

Turnout. Horses spend considerable time on pasture, and they need a safe environment and enough space to romp without crashing into something. One acre per horse with safe fencing is adequate. Deep holes should be filled and toxic plants or trees must be removed. If your turnout becomes flooded and your horse has no standing area out of the water, it may be wise not to use it. If there are no alternatives, keep the turnout short—no more than thirty to forty-five minutes. Hooves that are submerged in water too long become soft, causing the hoof's wall and lumen to separate, and abscesses or seedy toes may result. Hooves seem to be more

4

tolerant of mud, but deep, sucking mud can stress the legs, injure muscles, and pull off the horse's shoes.

Turning horses out on ice, especially when shod, is an open invitation to injury. They are subject to falling. Loss of balance or sliding can pull a muscle, or they can crash into a solid object.

Practice good riding habits and examine your horse's legs for any hot spots or lumps before and after working .

Never work a horse excessively for long periods of time or on hard surfaces. For example, steady jumping or barrel rac-

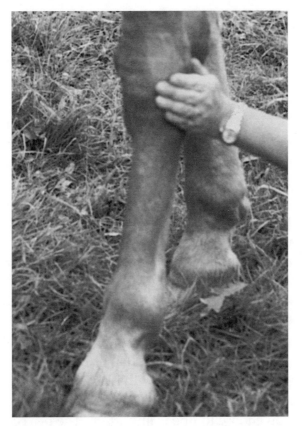

Hot spots are located by pressing the flat of the hand against the leg. All legs should be examined. When a warm spot is suspect, compare it with the same site on the opposite leg.

ing for more than twenty to twenty-five minutes without a rest is considered excessive. When horses have been worked long enough, they normally show fatigue and many exhibit a high body temperature, heavy breathing, and heavy sweating, which indicates they are ready to be walked out, cooled, and cared for.

Riding at a full gallop for long periods of time on the road as a daily ritual is conducive to sore feet and legs, because the road's hard surface is intended for automobiles that have air in their tires to cushion the ride. Many horsepeople ride or drive

---

Remember — if your horse has been idle,
condition him gradually.

---

their horses on the road. Where this type of condition persists or is necessary every day, have the farrier install heavy-duty concussion pads. These pads absorb the shock instead of the horse's legs and feet.

When clinics and shows are not attended often, excessive riding time may occur. During such times, remember to support your horse's legs with either bandages or good leg boots. Be alert for any limping. Soreness means your horse is through working and the show is over for now.

After each session the horse should be completely walked out, cooled, and relaxed by hosing, rinsing with liniment or a good brace, massaging, drying off, and then he should be put into standing wraps overnight. Upon returning home, he should be given a few days off to rest, with nightly leg wraps and only light exercise for at least a week.

Where you choose to ride is important. The perfect areas are, of course, a sand or Fibar ring and a rock free terrain. Grass is excellent cushioning, but wet grass can be slippery for iron shoes. Hard ground is tiring for a horse's legs when galloping, jumping, or working for long periods. Following such workouts, perhaps a fox hunt or cattle roundup, you should put your horse into standing wraps for the night after a good grooming and some liniment and massage. Rocky terrain is especially hard on a horse's feet and legs. An unshod horse can tear up his feet on rocks, and even if he is shod he can traumatize the joints, ligaments, and tendons.

Jumping on hard surfaces will invite splints and other stress problems.When arranging a jump course, be certain the horses are not coming off an obstacle onto a rock or extremely hard ground. Each side of a jump is generally raked and the footing loosened down 6 to 8 inches. When the ground within an outdoor course is softened at the landing sites by a disk or tiller, hidden rocks are often discovered and must be removed. If a large unremovable boulder is found, relocate the jump. During winter months, spread bedding several inches deep on both sides of the jump to soften landings and avoid slipping.

Be alert for any limping. Soreness means the clinic or show is over for the horse. Hot Spots on your horse's legs will be discerned during a leg check or "touch" examination. You may learn how to locate heat or hot spots by feeling of your horse's legs for excessively warm areas. If you feel a warm pastern or leg, compare it with the other leg. A hot spot will be much warmer than the rest of the limb or its opposite.

With these simple routines and suggestions in mind, you can do much to prevent injury. Now we can move on to the actual wrapping and bandaging that will also prolong the soundness of your horse's feet and legs.

Protective and Supportive Leg Coverings

All four of a young horse's legs should be protected with bandages or combination tendon/splint boots during longeing, breaking, and schooling. When polo bandages and/or boots are applied early in training, the horse's legs are cushioned against blows should he kick himself or lose his balance.

Any individual who is new to caring for a horse's legs might seek out a knowledgeable salesperson at a local tack shop when making their first purchases. Most bandage and quilt manufacturers identify the product, but not their use, on the package. They simply assume anyone making such a purchase is either experienced or will seek out some assistance.

There are knitted bandages, flannel or flannel-type, as well as a variety of weights and thicknesses of quilts. Each kind of bandage has a particular job to do.

Polo Bandages

Flannel polo bandages are used on all horses, but primarily when training begins and during schooling or exercising. Polos are used on hunters, jumpers, dressage horses, reining horses, driving, horses in competitive trail ride training, and all riding horses that have an interference problem. An older horse's legs can be protected with polos during workouts. Polos may be used on recovering lame horses during turnout. They are the easiest bandages to apply because they do not stretch, and come in bright or pastel colors as well as designer prints. Fashionable polos may be purchased, but the fancy designs will cost extra.

Track Bandages

Knitted track bandages are used over cotton sheets during training of race horses and, sometimes, jumpers. When properly applied, they give excellent support to hard-working legs. They are colorful and give the horse a "lift."

They may be used to substitute for regular standing bandages over quilts for either standing or shipping. However,

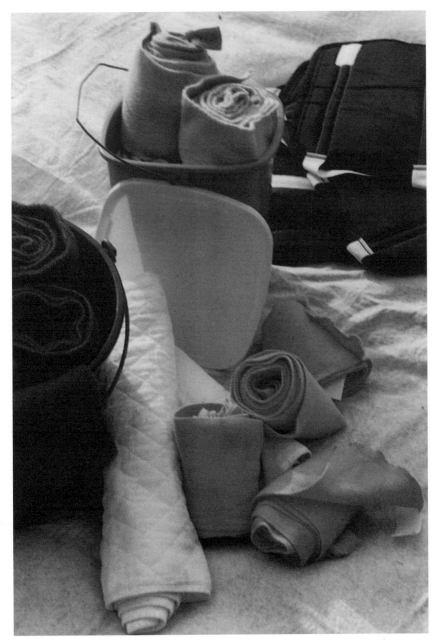

The many kinds of leg wraps and bandages kept in a riding stable or training barn. There are standing wraps, exercise and training bandages (polo wraps), cotton sheets, and quilts.

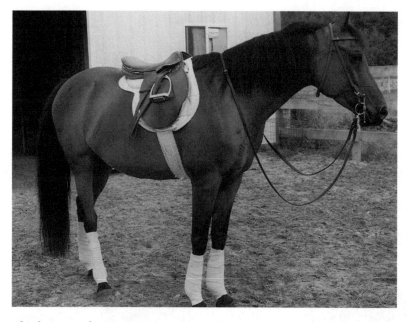

This horse, with polo bandages properly applied, is waiting for a workout.

they are narrow; therefore, when applied to a large horse they usually lack sufficient length. They work well over quilts on ponies, however.

Quilted Leg Wraps

Quilts are used for padding under bandages for shipping or for therapeutic purposes. Quilts come in lightweight, medium, and heavy. The heavy quilts are often referred to as pillow wraps. Regular cotton quilts come four to a package. The sizes range from twelve inches wide by twenty-six inches long to sixteen by thirty inches. The heavy, poly fiber pillow wraps have a cotton covering, and they are purchased in pairs. They can be sized to fit both front and rear legs.

Quilts and Bandages Together.

Wide, tightly knitted or flannel-type bandages are applied

over quilts and become support with padding for inactive or sore legs. This type of bandage/wrap is referred to as stall wraps, standing wraps, therapeutic wraps and sometimes night wraps. They are utilized when the horse is at rest. If wrapped low over the pastern, they act as shipping wraps during trailering or transporting. They are not used for exercising or working a horse.

Stall or Standing Bandages

Standing wraps are wide (usually five inches) and extra long (five to eight yards). They come knitted or in a flannel-type. They are used only *over* quilts for shipping or for therapeutic purposes. Flannel-type bandages are woven fabric, usually cotton or a blend with a light flannel on only one side. No fastener is included; therefore, masking tape is applied to hold them in place. They are reasonably priced and used for shipping or standing. The flannel is wrapped on the inside.

Elastic Bandages

Ace is a popular brand. These are an elastic knit bandage similar to the ones used by people, however, they are wrapped much differently. They may be somewhat wider and certainly longer. Lightweight quilts or rubberized sheets are wrapped on the legs, followed with the elastic bandage, which is wound over the quilt. Ace bandages should only be used by professional trainers. Racing trainers sometimes prefer them for trotting and pacing horses.

Cotton Leg Wrap Sheets

These disposable, seamless cotton sheets that measure thirty-by-thirty-six inches in size are folded before being placed on the horse's leg. One package contains from eight to twelve wraps, or they are available by the bale.

Bandaging Cotton

For veterinary use, cotton comes as a non-sterile roll of batten. The one-pound roll measures sixty-four inches in length and is about twelve inches in width.

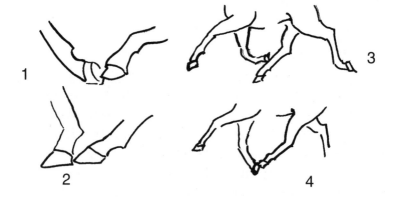

Interference: 1) forging, 2) over-reaching, 3) scalping, and 4) cross-firing. Cross-firing also occurs when both front or back feet rub or strike together during transit.

CHAPTER 2
Polo Wraps for Working Horses

Polos are often preferred for training because they offer twofold protection—support that aids undeveloped or tired muscles, especially during early training or after a lay-up, and padding. This cushioning prevents injuries such as skin scrapes caused by cross-firing, scalping, or overreaching, and raps made while jumping.

ROLLING BANDAGES

When you purchase a package of polos, you must prepare them for use. Manufacturers package the wraps to display them. They are rolled to show the type of fastener or how they will look after they have been applied to the horse's legs. Before using them, unroll, fold the end over, place the Velcro fasteners together, then roll. The Velcro should be on the outside for fastening upon completion of bandaging. It is important that you store the rolled bandages in a container to keep them clean until used.

If you like gadgets, tack suppliers offer a hand-driven bandage-rolling machine. It may be worth your looking into.

Preparing To Wrap Your Horse's Legs

Collect the bandages and grooming equipment needed before positioning your horse. Attempt to have everything ready so that your horse is not left standing alone (unless he is not disturbed when deserted).

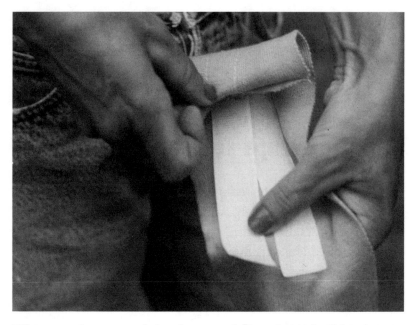

When you take a new polo bandage out of the package, the Velcro fastener tabs are on the outside. They must be re-rolled before applying. Fold and place the Velcro ends together as shown, then roll with these fasteners on the inside.

If wrapping is a new experience for the horse as well as for you, place him on cross-ties when the barn is quiet. Attempting to keep your horse's attention when other activities are going on is difficult, and showing a green horse something new and frightening in a busy aisle is impossible. Do not attempt wrapping when someone is feeding the other horses. Most horses are curious about any activity, and very young horses are distracted quickly.

If cross-ties or privacy are unavailable, find a safe, out-of-the-way location where you and your equine student can work without distractions. Set him up so that he cannot constantly move away from you. You may need a helper to hold him the first few times you wrap his legs.

The area must be level because the horse's weight must be

distributed evenly on all four feet. Never wrap a leg that is cocked. If he's not standing squarely, ask your horse to move over in order to shift weight onto the leg about to be wrapped.

If you are working outside, avoid weeds and high grass that will hinder your activity. Grass also invites your horse to eat. His attention should be on you, not on food. If you permit your horse to graze or eat hay, he will be moving constantly, making it nearly impossible to work on the legs.

Do not use a stall. Even though a stall is private and confining, you could be injured if the horse becomes excited. An oversized foaling stall, free of bedding, where you can tie your horse at one end may be suitable. Bedding poses a hazard because it can become caught in the bandage, causing a tendon problem. When a piece of something hard, such as

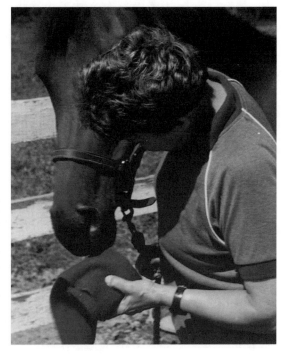

When your horse is inexperienced or excitable, go slowly and introduce new equipment before putting it on her. This will make your job easier and avoid an unwanted reaction.

a stick of hay or straw, dirt, or bedding rubs on or presses against the horse's leg for any length of time or while he's active, it can cause soreness or even a bowed tendon.

Be sure that your horse is not apprehensive about the equipment. If he has been wrapped previously, he should have little, if any, fear. Even so, show a bandage to him and allow him to see and smell what is going to be placed on his legs. Use this opportunity to roll the bandages. Let the young horse watch and sniff.

Before you apply wraps, your horse's legs must be free of dirt and debris. Do not wear gloves because you must feel the legs for grit, scabs, or bumps. During and after brushing, a thorough check with the fingers will also disclose any "hot spots" that indicate trauma. If you find a hot spot on a leg or foot, give it immediate attention and postpone working the horse. After working, always check the legs again for any trauma or injury before you put your horse away. (Chapter 6 discusses injuries and hot spots and what you should do for them.)

Once you have prepared all four bandages and your horse's legs have been brushed and cleaned thoroughly, the job of wrapping begins.

APPLYING A POLO BANDAGE

It is very important to wind the bandage in the proper direction on the leg. The horse's legs are delicate, and winding from the inside out gives the legs ample support without binding the tendons. Please note the diagram on the following page.

Do not wear gloves because you will not be able to feel through the fabric with the tips of your fingers. It is important to feel how the bandage is lying against the leg. Keep your

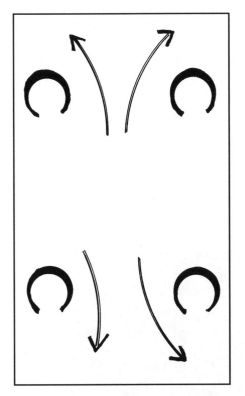

Always wind bandages or sheets in the direction indicated here.

fingers free to detect any wrinkles or twists.

Start wrapping at the cannon bone, just below the knee. If you are right-handed, hold the tip of the bandage in place with your left hand while you bring the roll out between your horse's legs. Continue to hold the end in place until you have made the first wrap. Then begin to wind downward at about one-and-one-half-inch intervals. If you leave the tip of the bandage high, you can place a finger on it to keep the bandage from moving. Watch carefully for foreign matter sticking to the wrap.

Maintain constant tension so that the bandage is secure without being too tight. (Study the step-by-step illustrations.) The wrapping job must NOT be tight at the top and loose at the bottom, or vice-versa. If you believe the tension is mixed—loose and tight—start over. To check for tightness, try to insert a finger inside the top and bottom of the bandage. If one finger can be inserted, the tension is fine, but if two fingers can be inserted, the wrap is too loose.

If your wrap is consistently too loose, practice firming up as you wind. To firm up the tension while winding to create a supportive wrap that will not bind, secure the bandage across the front of the leg (over the cannon bone) with a very gentle tug. Be scrupulous in doing this! NEVER PULL THE BANDAGE TIGHTLY ACROSS THE BACK OF THE LEG

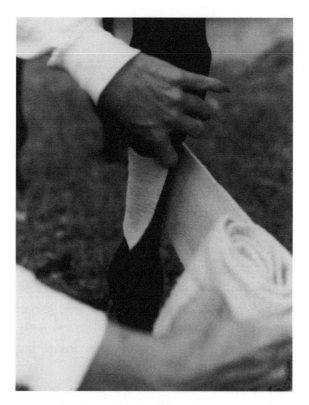

Start the polo wrap in front at the canon bone. As you begin to wrap, hold the tip of the bandage down with one finger to prevent it from slipping.

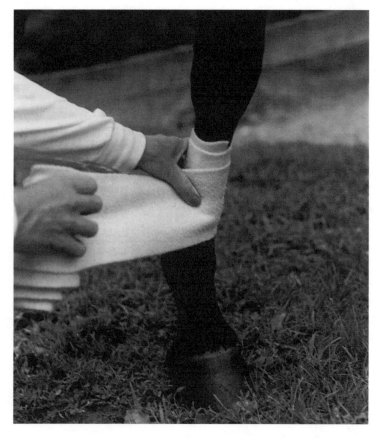

After a couple of winds have been made, it should not be necessary to hold the corner in place. If the wrapping slips, it is too loose. Wind downward at two-inch spacing for most wraps, or one-and-one-half-inch intervals for a horse that interferes.

where a tendon is located, but rather roll it securely around behind. Now check that it is notoo tight or pulled.

To protect the fetlock and upper pastern area, wind the bandage over the fetlock and ankle. From the front, wrap around the ankle behind and downward, then aim upward as you wind across the front to make a "V." Making this crossover at the front of the ankle frees the foot for easier flexion.

To cover the fetlock, aim downward and wap behind and under, then bring the bandage up toward the front of the leg.

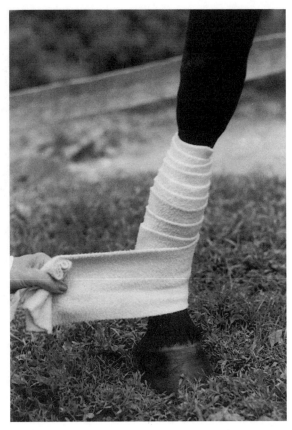

Now, wrap the bandage upward with the spacing between the winds wider apart. If you reach the top and have bandage left over, which is not likely, DO NOT WIND DOWNWARD. Wrap around the top again below the knee. The Velcro fasteners should end up on the front or outside of the leg where they cannot be accidentally kicked loose.

Check Your Wrappings

When finished, check all of your wrappings on all legs. Check for even tension (any sagging or tight spots), for any binding or "wrinkles," and for a too-loose or too-tight bandage. Remember to insert a finger down inside each

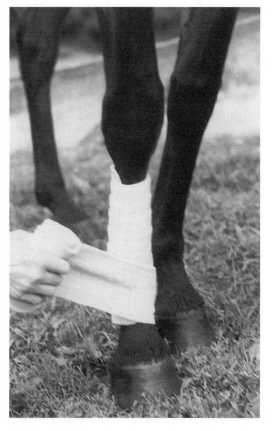

Cross the bandage over the front of the pastern and wind upward, creating a "V" where the ankle joint bends. When you reach the top, finish the wind. *Do not* start downward again.

bandage. If you are going to ride, be certain that the fasteners cannot be kicked loose. Finally, be sure that the wrap is low enough under the fetlock to protect it if necessary. The fetlock and pastern area are covered during early training and where there is interference from other feet.

When your horse will be ridden in the polo wraps, always use extra precautions with fasteners. When you are topside you cannot see what is happening around your horse's legs should a bandage come undone. This rule is often partially relaxed by some handlers when the horse is not to be ridden and is quiet on the longe line.

I learned a lesson about checking bandages from an incident at a riding school several years ago. A student had rushed to prepare her young horse for schooling. While she worked the colt in the ring at a fast warm-up trot, a bandage on one of the colt's front legs came loose and began to unravel just as she asked him for a half-turn. The opposite leg became entangled, the horse lost its balance, and they both fell. Generally, when a bandage comes undone, all that results is a torn bandage. In this case, however, the colt panicked and tried to escape the "trap" that he felt on his leg.

Always ask yourself, "Does it look like a good wrapping job?" Never be hesitant about rewrapping. In fact, when you are first learning, you will need to rewrap often. After you have been doing it for ten or fifteen years, you still need to

Test the wrapping to see if it is too loose or too tight by sliding a finger under the top of it. Your finger should slide underneath without difficulty, and the wrap should feel snug.

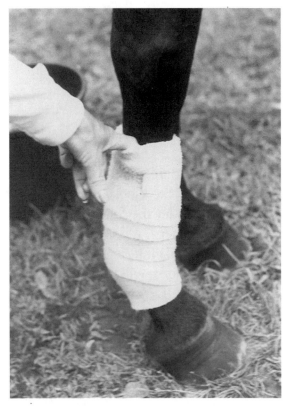

rewrap on occasion. Never attempt to salvage a poor wrap-ping job!

WHEN TO GO UNWRAPPED

Once the green horse is beginning to school well and is not interfering, light work without wraps may occasionally be advisable, such as a fifteen-minute walk and trot, especially if he is kept in a barn with infrequent turnout. It is important to avoid small circling the first few times. The reason for briefly going unwrapped is to permit the young horse's legs to become less dependent upon the support furnished by wraps. Horses that are turned out all day and have romping space seldom need this type of exercise. Long walks under saddle without the support of wraps will strengthen

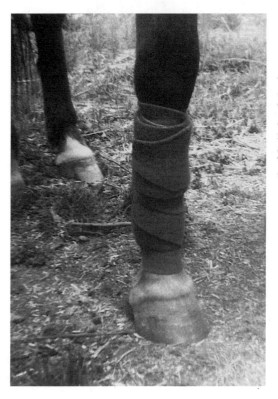

This is a typical first-time wrapping job. The winds are loose and irregular, with most of the wrap around the top. The student had to do these wraps over.

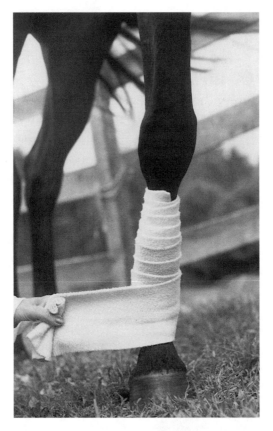

Applying a polo wrap to a horse that interferes. The bandage is wrapped for thickness, and to protect the lower leg and fetlock from bruises and scrapes.

any young horse's legs. If, however, the horse is inclined to interfere, it is best to wait until his strides are balanced before you begin this practice.

CLEANING AND CARE OF BANDAGES

Maintaining clean and repaired training equipment is essential in a working barn. Anyone who works around horses knows only too well that time around the horses passes very quickly because of endless chores. Training time may begin sooner if the bandages and tack are clean and ready to use when the horse is put on cross-ties.

Washing Suggestions

Cleanliness and maintenance of horse equipment are important unless you can afford to replace it often. Gentle but thorough cleaning methods are recommended. Observe these precautions during washing.

Cleaning Agents. Be careful with the kind of soaps and cleaning agents used on your horse's equipment. There are a few tough-hide-type horses that do not seem to be bothered with skin irritants, but most are very sensitive, especially to harsh soaps and detergents. The safest cleaning agents for equipment of skin-sensitive horses are washing soda or Ivory soap. Use one tablespoon of washing soda or Ivory soap for each set of bandages. Wash them in cold water. If quilts and dirty saddle pads are added to the wash, especially if they are covered with sweaty dirt, you may need to add two ounces of washing soda to the load. If the quilts are badly stained, add two or three tablespoons of chlorine bleach to the water before you put in any items. Chlorine also sanitizes, especially if fungus is infesting your horse's legs. Saddle pads may be treated this way, also. Always rinse completely, and use lots of cold water.

Machine Washing. The long, narrow strips of bandages tend to wind and become knotted when washed in the family washer. To avoid tight tangles and tearing, try one of the following methods:

• Use a gentle cycle. Mix in quilts and towels or a couple of saddle pads to discourage tangling.

• Stuff the bandages into pillowcases or washing bags. Close them with safety pins if necessary. If you are washing polo bandages, put one pair per bag so as not to crowd them. The object is to keep them from twisting. Packing them loosely in bags also permits tangling, so it is important that you close the bags sufficiently.

Hand Washing. Around the barn, a quick washing usually is done by hand. To remove the excess water, squeeze the quilts and bandages—do not wring or twist them. Polos tend to lose their soft cushioning flannel when washed many times in machines. Hand washing will keep them fluffy longer.

A bandage-washing machine that can be used in the barn or stable is available. It apparently has a very gentle cycle that does not whip the ends into tangles and knots nor does it pull much of the soft flannel out of the weave. The bandage washer is available through horse-equipment vendors.

Drying Bandages. To dry polos without stretching them out of shape, after you wash the bandages, fold the strips in half and hang each end over a line or rack to dry. Distributing the weight, prevents the fabric from being stretched. You can place clothespins between the bandages to keep them from sliding, but do not use them to hold the bandages. You can also hang them over plastic hangers when space is short.

Storing Bandages

Locate the proper-sized container that will hold a complete set of bandages. If you use the bandages every day, you may want to keep them in a pail or caddy. If you have more than one set, store the freshly cleaned ones in a trunk or closed container that will keep out dust and pieces of hay. Bandages and quilts that are used infrequently are stored in a caddy or bucket, and any that are not quite clean should be kept away from dusty areas and where there is bedding or hay. Polo bandages are flannel and will collect trash.

Plastic bags with handles from the grocery store are convenient for storage. The handles can be tied together to close

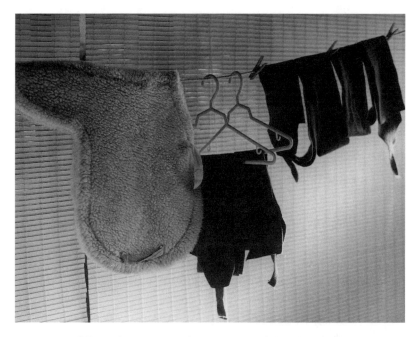

Mixing a saddle pad or some quilt wraps in with bandages when washing them in a machine will lessen tangling. When hanging them to dry, always fold the wet bandages so the weight of the water does not stretch them out of shape.

the bag as well as act as hangers. The bags are large enough to accommodate a set of standing wraps and quilts or a set of polos. They may be hung from a tack hook or kept on shelves or inside a trunk. Another possible storage container for a set of bandages could be a five- or seven-pound size feed supplement container. Bandage racks are available that may be hung in the tack room or on the side of a trunk. The wire-basket type of bandage containers are great when hung on the outside of the trunk or portable stall at a show.

Bandages are often damp from sweat or wet ground after your horse works out. If they are still clean enough to use again, hang them up to dry on a fence, a blanket rack, or a line stretched across an open area.

Helpful Tips

• To make your first attempts at wrapping easier, set aside a few practice sessions just prior to working your horse. A patient, sleepy-type horse makes the best subject for practicing until you become proficient.

• Remember to pick out the hooves before bandaging the legs because the horse's ankles will be more flexible before they are covered.

• Tie up the tail before bandaging the rear legs to keep the hair from interfering with your wraps.

• During fly season, always apply a fly repellent on your horse first.

CHAPTER 3

Track Bandages for Sporting Horses

Track or exercise bandages are excellent leg support for horses that are in vigorous training, such as racing, jumping, eventing, or steeplechase. This type of bandage, however, is best used only by knowledgeable and trained hands.

The difference between track/exercise bandages and polos is that track bandages stretch more with the leg's action while providing very secure support. They hug the legs so that the horse feels a supportive "lift." Track bandages come in varying lengths and elasticity for greater or lesser support. Because of this elastic effect, however, track bandages can bind on the legs. Therefore, a barrier (sheeting) is applied first to prevent the edges of the bandage from pressing on or cutting into the horse's tendons. Sheeting is typically made of cotton and is disposable.

You must wrap track bandages with great care and they are not easy to apply. If you wrap these bandages incorrectly or too tightly, the horse's legs may swell, disabling him for several days or longer. If loosely wrapped, they give no support to the legs.

Horsemanship students and working students in stables or at race tracks need to learn how to use exercise/track and

Ace bandages. Until you become proficient with stall wraps and polos, however, it is wise to postpone any attempts with track or Ace bandages. I strongly suggest that your trainer or teacher also check the bandages before you work the horse.

What happens if a stretch-type or elastic bandage edge **binds on a leg** during a workout, or afterward while the horse is cooling down? Binding shuts off the circulation and the leg begins to swell. If this happens, you must quickly remove the wrap and hose the leg with cold water immediately to reduce swelling. If you don't unwrap the leg in time it can swell to twice its size (called cording) and make the horse lame.

Trotter and pacer trainers use elastic or Ace bandages with special lightweight cotton quilts or rubberized sheets as a liner wrap. The wrapping procedure for elastic or Ace bandages is the same as for track bandages. The racing seasons require horses to practice on tracks that are often frozen and hard while preparing for early spring meets. Two-year-old Standardbreds starting in training for spring racing as trotters or pacers benefit from the support that these types of bandages give their tender, often underdeveloped, legs.

Correct Wrapping Directions. Wrap from the center out between the legs. The arrows indicate the direction to wrap around each leg.

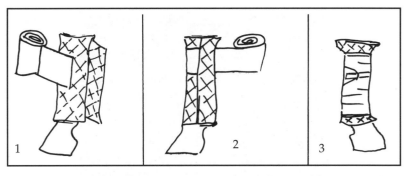

The knitted bandage is wrapped over the cotton sheet in the same winding manner as with standing wraps or polos. 1) Start the bandage at the front with the end under the edge of the quilt. 2)Roll the bandage around near the top. Do not pull. 3) Upon reaching the fetlock, start back up the leg. The fastener must be on the outside or front where the horse cannot kick it loose.

HOW TO WRAP TRACK BANDAGES

The following instructions are offered for individuals or students in equine schools or under the guidance of a professional trainer. If you haven't done so already, seriously consider practicing with standing bandages and polo bandages before starting with these more difficult wraps.

Applying the Sheets

When you are applying a cotton sheet, begin wrapping from the center outward between the legs. The sheeting must be wrapped closely and as smoothly as possible on the leg. Do not permit any deep wrinkles. (Refer to the figure above for applying the cotton sheet and bandages and to the previous page for correct winding directions.)

When the cotton sheet is in place, insert the end of the bandage under the edge of the sheet with the end over the cannon bone. Be certain that at least one inch of sheet is protruding at the top. Wind the bandage down the leg at about one-and-one-half-inch intervals, using the same technique as you use for wrapping polos. Be sure to keep an even tension,

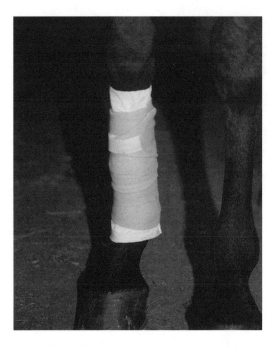

Notice how the sheet protrudes over and below
the track bandage to prevent it from cutting into
the leg.

and do not permit the bandage to wrinkle. Keep it smooth
and use your fingers to check it.

Wrapping with correct tension takes considerable practice. These bandages will sag if they are wrapped loosely and
will offer no support whatsoever. You can avoid winding
them too loosely by securing the winds over the cannon bone
at each go-around. On the other hand, the bandage will
pinch if it is too tight. You can avoid wrapping too tightly by
not pulling and stretching the bandage on the leg.

At the ankle, you have the option of covering or not covering under the fetlock. Because track bandages do not offer
any padding effect, the only reason for wrapping under is to
support the sesamoid area. When you wrap this low, be certain that enough sheet is protruding at the bottom to shield

the bare leg from the bandage. If covering the fetlock, and the sheeting covers low enough, make a "V" over the front (as you would with polos), then wrap upward. If bandage is left over when you reach the knee or hock, do not wrap downward. Continue around the top until the bandage is fastened.

If enough bandage is left over to wrap around the top a few times, check for a too-tight bandage! Unwrap and start over. Unless you are wrapping a small pony, you may have pulled the bandage too tight or made the winds too far apart. The bandage should be distributed evenly throughout the wrapped leg. When you are finished, double-check to see that an inch or so of sheeting is visible at both top and bottom to prevent cording. Then insert your finger to check for tightness.

WHEN TO USE FRESH SHEETS

A package of sheeting usually contains eight to twelve wraps. The sheets may be reused a time or two if they do not become torn or soiled. When they are soiled, torn, or badly wrinkled, pull out a fresh, new one. Most racing trainers use fresh sheets each time a horse does track work, and some use double sheets. It is costly to use up a ten-to-twelve-dollar package of sheeting every few days, but, compared to maintaining the soundness of a colt valued at $6,000 or more, this can hardly be considered a waste.

NEVER LEAVE A HORSE STANDING IN TRACK BANDAGES. Leaving a horse standing in track bandages invites leg problems. Horses left unattended may cord up and become lame for several weeks. At some training and racing stables, horses are sometimes left unattended after a workout because everyone is extremely busy. This practice is harmful to the horses and costly to owners. It takes less than two minutes to remove a set of wraps! Horses that are hot walked should be unwrapped when they are removed from the walker. Horses that are hand walked may be unwrapped during untacking.

Never wrap a horse and then leave him in his stall until he is worked. The horse's legs should be wrapped just prior to a workout.

CHAPTER 4
Standing Wraps

Standing wraps are exactly what their name implies. They are often referred to as stall wraps, therapeutic wraps, pressure bandages, and night wraps. When applied low on the horse's legs to cover the coronary band they function as shipping wraps. Standing wraps are quilts, although you may use substitute materials in an emergency.

WHEN TO USE STANDING WRAPS

Standing wraps are important when your horse is over tired, sore, or laid-up. If you exhibit, fox hunt, or cut cattle with your horse, it is a good idea to apply night wraps to rest and soothe his legs. After a hard workout when your horse is tired or a little sore, wrapping his legs is the humane thing to do. Nighttime wraps when your horse has been exerted help keep his limbs sound.

During stall-bound periods, you can also use wraps to prevent stocking-up. Frequently, back legs will swell during a confining lay-up if they are not wrapped nightly. Swelling occurs because of poor circulation in the horse's back legs, and mares are particularly susceptible. Hand walking or an hour of quiet turnout will reduce swelling, but if walking or turnout is not possible, you must apply wraps.

When you are treating a sore foot or leg, wrap all four legs because the horse will shift his weight to rest the supporting limb. The opposite, uninjured legs sustain the most weight because your horse shifts away from the pain. Therefore, both front and back legs must be wrapped, because the unimpaired opposite legs need supplemental support to prevent fatigue-stress.

SCHEDULES FOR USING

Standing wraps are left on overnight or during a rest period for twelve or fewer hours. Your veterinarian may occasionally prescribe around-the-clock-wraps. Twenty-four-hour wrapping is based on a twelve-hour schedule, which means that the legs are thoroughly brushed down and re-wrapped in the morning and again in the evening.

Where therapy is involved, seek your veterinarian's advice regarding a good schedule. For example, if you are using cold therapy or applying a poultice, you must rewrap

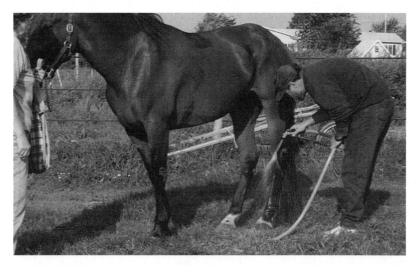

After a training session, this Standardbred's legs are being hosed with cold water. Afterward he will be placed in standing wraps. Cold wet wraps might also be applied.

the legs after the morning feeding, then again before closing up the barn for the night. You also rewrap the legs after each therapy session.

Leaving wraps in place for more than twelve hours can cause leg problems. Horses are heavy animals and when they move around the bandages are disturbed. A wrap can slip or twist, or foreign matter such as bedding may work its way underneath the wrap. A tendon injury, sometimes referred to as a bandage bow (bowed tendon), may develop because a wrap has been left on too long, or cording can occur. In any case, when the legs are unwrapped and brushed, they have an opportunity to "breathe," encouraging much-needed circulation.

APPLYING A STANDING BANDAGE

As discussed previously, always groom your horse before you apply bandages. *Cleanliness* is paramount. Brush down the legs thoroughly. Remove any grit or other foreign matter that might rub against a leg, and pick the feet prior to wrapping. Be careful to keep the bandages from coming into contact with the ground where they will pick up dirt.

Quilt sizes

The usual quilt widths (length of the cannon bone) are twelve or fourteen inches. A longer width (sixteen inches) for a larger horse or for shipping-wrap use is available. Horses over fifteen hands will likely use the fourteen-inch size. Some Thoroughbred and Warmblood trainers use twelve-inch quilts on the front legs and fourteen-inch on the rear legs. For small horses and ponies, the quilt is sometimes folded to shorten it to the correct length. Be sure that the edge is not wrapped against the leg. Your objective is to provide protection and support over as much of the lower leg as possible,

The quilt may be folded over at the top to fit small horses and ponies. The edge of the quilt must be on the outside so it does not rub.

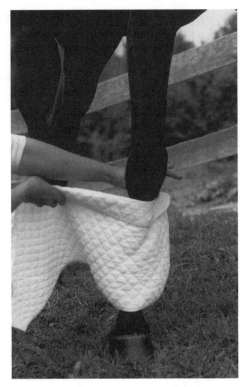

and sometimes down over the pastern. This means that "too large is better than too small."

Wrapping

Start the quilt by holding the edge on the front of the leg. Wrap from the center outward, between the horse's legs. (Refer to the illustrations for a better understanding of this task.) Keep the wrap smooth against the horse's leg. You do not want any creases or quilt edges rubbing against a tendon.

When you are wrapping for therapeutic purposes, the quilt should reach from the knee down to the ankle, but do not allow it to touch the ground or it will act as a wick and absorb any dampness it contacts from the stall bedding. If the quilt is a bit too long, it is better to let it protrude over the

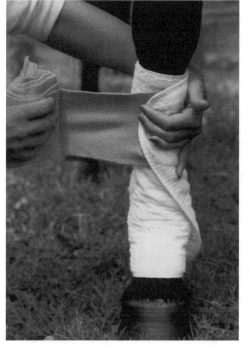

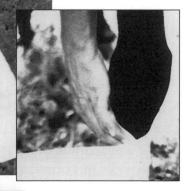

To begin a standing wrap, hold the seam of the quilt at the inside of theleg and wrap from the center out, between the legs.

Hold the front of the quilt in place so it cannot slip as you wind. Keep the quilt smooth against the horse's leg.

Insert the end of the bandage under the edge of the quilt at the front of the leg. Hold the end in place until you have made the first complete wrap around the leg.

knee or hock. Just be careful that you begin winding the *bandage* below the hock or knee joint.

If your wrapped quilt ends at or near the front of the leg (where it should), insert the end of the bandage under the edge. This is at a point below the front of the knee, on the cannon bone. Be certain that the rolled bandage is turned so that it will unroll as you wind around the leg.

Start by winding to the back. Continue in the same direction over the quilt, leaving plenty of quilt wrap showing at the top. When the bandage has been secured with the first go-around over the quilted wrap, the job becomes easier. Continue to hold the end in place until the first wrap has been made so that the quilt does not slip around the leg and lose its position.

Now aim downward, with your next winds at approximately one-and-one-half-inch intervals, covering the quilt evenly. Take your time and smooth out any wrinkles.

Learn to wrap evenly and snugly. A loose bandage is of no value. Wrap so that the bandage will stay in place and support the leg. Until you are able to wrap securely, you might try wrapping the bandage snugly across the front of the leg (the cannon bone), then wind it behind. DO NOT TUG THE BANDAGE across the back of the leg where the tendon is located, and DO NOT STRETCH the bandage around the leg, because this will make it too tight. You do not want to impede circulation. Be advised that leg trauma will result if a bandage is twisted or applied too tightly. It will also happen if the quilt is not beneath the bandage. The direction in which you wrap is especially important in order to avoid further tension on the tendons. (See chart on page 17.)

Maintain an even tension throughout; in other words, if you see that the top is loose, do not wind the rest of the leg tighter to compensate. Undo it and start wrapping over again. Always rewrap the leg when you see a problem.

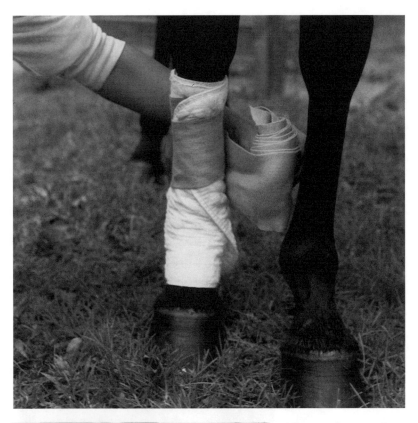

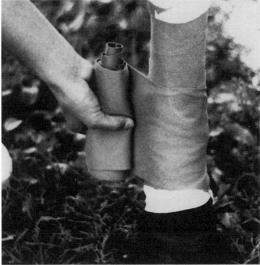

After you have made the first wind, aim downward at 1 1/2 to 2-inch intervals, covering the quilt evenly.

Cross over in front of the ankle and wind upward until you reach the knee or hock. If some bandage is left over, wrap it around at the top, taking care that it does not touch the leg. DO NOT WRAP BACK DOWN THE LEG. Fasteners must be in front or on the outside of the leg.

Wrapping for tired legs generally involves only the area from the knee or hock to the fetlock or ankle. If the area below the fetlock needs to be covered, be certain that the quilt is low enough before you wind down over and behind the joint.

To cover the fetlock, maintain proper, even tension as you wind behind, then upward in front. There should be a criss-cross over the front of the ankle. Continue to wrap upward with the spacing wider apart.

As you complete the wrap, your bandage may not end at the knee unless it is an extra-long type. At any rate, if excess remains, DO NOT START DOWNWARD AGAIN. Continue wrapping around the top to use up the rest of the ban-

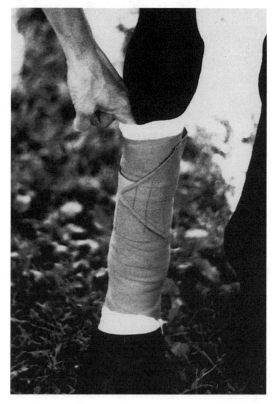

When completed, test the tension of the wrap. You should be able to insert a finger down inside the wrapping. The quilt should be exposed for one or two inches at both the top and bottom of the wrap.

dage. The Velcro fasteners should be either on the front or the outside of the leg so that they cannot be kicked off.

Check your work.

Now stand back and check your work. Is the tension even? Is there at least an inch or more of quilt above and below the bandage? You should be able to insert a finger comfortably but snugly down inside the wrapping.

Fasteners

Occasionally a set of standing bandages comes with ties instead of Velcro fasteners. Some inexpensive bandages have no fasteners at all and must be closed with masking tape cut approximately fourteen to eighteen inches in length. One- or two-inch masking tape made of paper will not bind. It may be wrapped completely around, holding the end of the bandage in place, and then wind upwards.

With ties, please use caution. Tie on the outside in bow knots that will stay in place, then tuck the ends of the strings inside the outer bandage. Masking tape may be applied for additional security.

EMERGENCY SUBSTITUTIONS FOR STANDING BANDAGES

When a new horse comes up sore and you haven't yet bought standing bandages, and the tack shop is closed, you can temporarily substitute one-inch-thick cotton batting fresh from the package. Another emergency substitute for quilts is a plain baby diaper. Be careful that no binding, bunching, or seams are present at the backs of the legs, no matter what material you use. Apply the material as smoothly as possible around the leg at least three or four times and cover it sufficiently so that the bandages do not make contact with the leg. Do not mix the kinds of substitutes. Both legs, whether front or back, must be wrapped equally.

The standing bandages themselves can be substituted with any fabric-type, non-elastic bandage, such as track bandages, polos, or shipping bandages, as long as there is adequate, smooth padding underneath. One enterprising horseman, a medical student, used tubular bandages from the emergency hospital room over pillow wraps after a show. These are available from a medical supply store and are four to six inches wide, when flattened, by at least twelve yards long. Do not use polos alone for overnight standing. They must be applied over a substantial liner or quilt wrap.

It is not a good idea to use one set of polos for a variety of needs. Polos are flannel and collect foreign material, and they are difficult to keep clean. They probably will require washing before being used to work the horse, and too many washings wear them out quickly. Polo bandages are generally not long enough to wrap over thick quilts on fourteen to sixteen inch legs. On the other hand, polo bandages that are too worn and have lost most of their flannel padding may be used with standing wraps on medium and small breeds of horses.

SHIPPING WRAPS

The same technique for wrapping stall or standing bandages apply to shipping wraps, except that the wrap should drop down over the pastern to protect the coronet band. If your quilts are not long enough to do this, your horse should wear bell boots, (see Chapter 5).

Take additional precautions with fastening. If a bandage comes off during transit your horse's feet can become entangled, especially during unloading, and he may panic. Masking tape placed around the top will reinforce and secure the fastening.

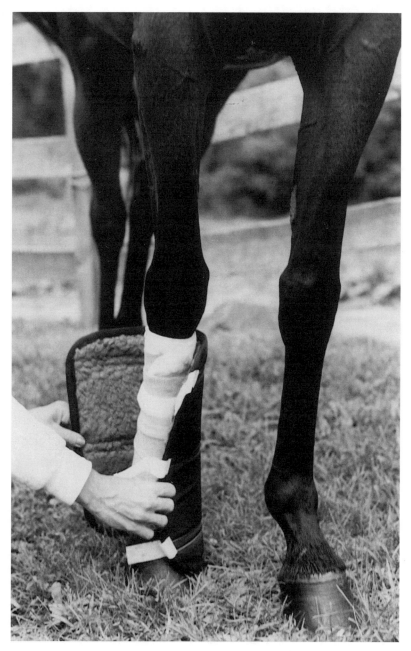

A square shipping wrap may be applied low over standing wraps to protect the coronet and provide additional padding.

Quilted-type shipping boots are frequently sized "short." They, too, must be supplemented with bell boots to cover the pastern and coronet. An injury to the coronet can lead to a long lay-up.

Young horses bounce around and easily become frightened. Their feet seem to fly in all directions at once. After applying shipping wraps on these horses, you can cover them with additional padding. Shipping squares are plain quilted boots with Velcro fasteners. The lower end of these boots may be applied low to cover the pastern area of each foot after bell boots have been put in place.

At journey's end remember to remove all the shipping wraps as soon as possible. It may be a good idea to re-roll them so they will stay clean and conveniently handy for application prior to the drive home, or for the next trip.

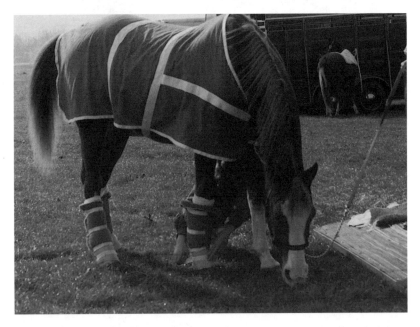

One variety of padded shipping boots. Velcro fasteners provide easy application and removal.

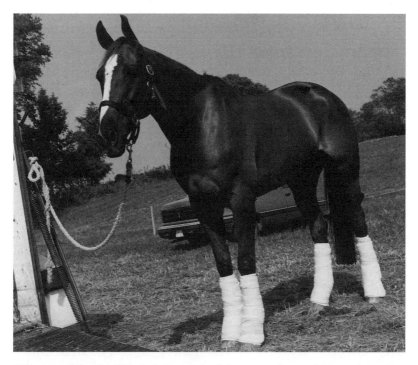

This warmblood gelding was prepared for a trip home from a show. His owner used medical tubular bandages over pillow wraps. The bandages were secure and supported his legs during a fourteen-hour trailer ride. *Sue A. Allen photo, reprinted from Horse and Horsemen.*

Cross Country and International Shipping

If you have your horse shipped by a professional transport service, a dispatcher should explain to you the procedure they follow for shipping horses over a period of days, as well as what their insurance covers. When your horse is hauled longer than twelve or fourteen hours, it is advisable to use shipping boots instead of bandages. Long-haul drivers frequently do not want the horses in bandages. Most commercial van operators will not rewrap bandages or replace boots on your horse's legs for you. If a boot comes off, it stays off. Inquire of your driver.

APPLYING COLD, WET WRAPS

These wraps are usually used on a horse that is not feeling his best. Before you stand him on ties, prepare your equipment. Just as you would for any other kind of wrap, select a good brush, a hoof pick, your quilts and bandages, and for this task, a small pail of very cold water.

Place the quilt(s) in the cold water to soak while you are grooming, or leave them at least long enough to thoroughly wet them. The wraps are applied to the legs soaking wet after some of the water has been gently squeezed out to avoid excessive dripping. Applying a wet quilt is the same as applying a standing wrap. This type of wrapping is left in place for twelve hours or less, while your horse relaxes in his stall, of course.

Ready-made products are available for cold wrapping, but unless ice is required, the cold, wet quilts work nicely. They are easy to keep clean by merely rinsing them out after each use and washing them occasionally. A barn with two horses requires only a couple sets of quilts and bandages for several kinds of chores. (See Chapter 6 for additional discussion of cold therapy.)

CHAPTER 5
Boots for
Working Horses

Boots provide protective support and padding for a working horse's legs. Many varieties are available, and each type suits a particular need. For example, padded boots soften the hard knocks that occur on high jump rails or from interference of another foot. Reining horses need protection on the hind fetlocks (sesamoid) from fast stops and spinning turns. The physiology of young or out-of-condition legs requires yet a different kind of support. Many trainers, both English and Western, use splint or tendon boots, or combination boots, on young show horses—and, of course, bandages or wraps.

Horse boots are available in a multitude of materials and colors. In addition to soft leather, stiff leather, and combinations, you will find boots made of neoprene, vinyl with lightweight padded liners, and fitted ready-wraps made of vinyl or other flexible materials. Splint and tendon boots constructed of a high grade leather or pigskin exterior with soft leather liners tend to wear for many years when given proper care. While the lightweight ready-wraps manufactured for the working horse's legs, joints, and feet are easy to install and keep clean, they do not wear or offer support for as long a period before needing replacement.

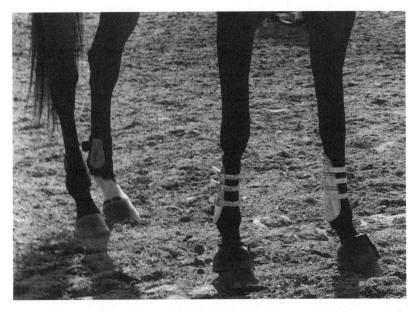

This Jumper Division Thoroughbred's legs and pasterns are well protected. He is wearing both open front tendon boots and bell boots in front, and ankle boots on the rear legs.

Bootmakers and inventors are becoming more and more conscious of the care a horse's legs require. Many performance horses today are put through rigorous work. Suppliers have produced some excellent protection for a horse's legs during competition or while recuperating from trauma. One brand, called the Sports Medicine Boot, is an energy absorber. In 1991, this boot was used immediately after a horse blew a tendon during competition. After being examined by two veterinarians, the horse continued to compete wearing Sports Medicine Boots and won. Most horsepeople would place an animal with such an injury into an ice boot and trailer him home.

A similar type of boot, Tough Glove Competition Boots, made by Sporthorse Equipment, is also an energy absorber with excellent impact deflection. In other words, the boots absorb concussive jolts.

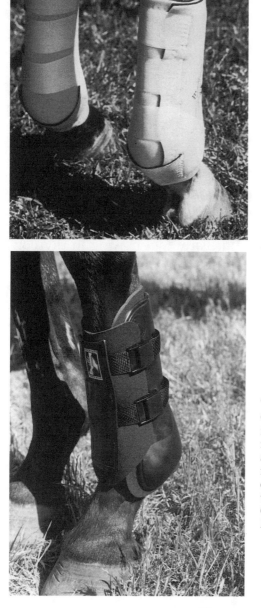

The Sports Medicine Boot, according to manufacturer Dr. C. N. Kobluk, is a valuable tool to prevent lower limb injuries during training and performance. The boot provides very high levels of energy absorption, which helps during rehabilitation of lower leg injury.
Courtesy of Professional's Choice Sports Medicine Products, Inc.

The Tough Glove Competition Boot with front panel which is removable. These boots are shock absorbing and retain a molded shape for excellent fit on the horse's legs.
Courtesy of Sporthorse Equipment.

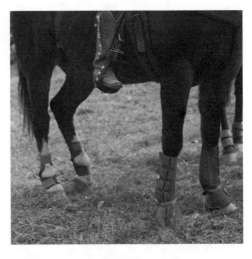

Combination skid boots on the rear and splint boots with pastern protection on the front. These fabric boots are popular with gymkhana exhibitors.

BOOTS AS AN ALTERNATIVE TO BANDAGES

You can use boots on performance horses when bandaging is not permitted, particularly for showing in divisions that physically stress the legs. There are still a few officiators at horse shows who will not permit bandages because there is a possibility of a wrap coming undone during competition. When a bandage unravels, it may become entangled around a foot and cause a bad fall. On the other hand, you see horses in training, in novice classes, and on the race track fully bandaged!

An experienced wrapper can bandage a horse's legs about as quickly as it takes to carefully buckle on boots (except for the boots with hook and loop closures). Time spent re-rolling bandages for the next use would replace the cleanup time necessary for the boots. You must also keep the bandages clean, but unless you work your horse in mud or wet grass, you can use the bandages a few times between washings. Merely shake any sand or dirt out and allow them to dry before you re-roll them. Expensive boots must be carefully cleaned and oiled after being used in wet conditions.

A young horse or a horse that is worked hard needs leg support and protection, and if you have never learned how to wrap, use the proper boots. Take great care that your horse's boots fit well. They must be neither too tight nor too loose and must cover the leg properly. Ill-fitting boots can cause as many problems as a poor wrapping job. It may be necessary to have the boots custom fit in order to obtain adequate support for a particular horse's legs. It is very important that the boots do not shift while your horse is working. They must fit and stay put. Also, be certain that the boots give the necessary support and pad your horse's legs well.

Another alternative is to obtain a good pair of ready-wraps. There are Hampa, Neoprene, Ulster International, Bandagetten and other brands that have Velcro or combination fasteners.

TYPES OF WORKING BOOTS

Splint boots are used on young jumpers, hunters, and reining or stock horses when leg support (splint protection) is required. A good pair will have a tough, cushioned patch to protect the inside splint bone.

Tendon boots are for jumpers or hunters. They are constructed to protect the tendons and are available with an open front that frees the leg's flexibility and lightens the weight of the boots. Open fronts, however, do not provide any cushioning for the front of the legs.

Tendon and splint boots combined often include protection for the ankle and may be purchased for either front or hind legs. They have an inside reinforcement (often rubber) for tendon support and protection. A leather patch covers the inside splint and ankle.

Tendon boots that provide support, protection against impact, and that can be used during trauma recovery are now

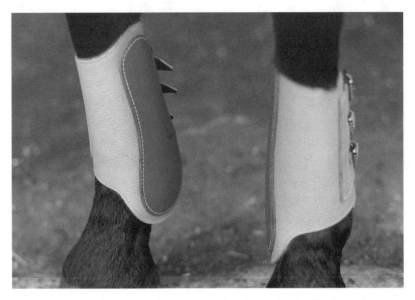

A pair of pigskin tendon/splint combination boots for the forelegs are an investment. They look great and wear for a long time. They are lined with soft rubber to provide padding.

coming onto the market. Tests results are favorable, and performance horses may benefit greatly from the shock absorbing capability of these boots. They are manufactured from materials that are lightweight and that mold to the legs for correct fit, which means no slipping.

Skid boots, sometimes referred to as **run down** or **sesamoid boots**, are worn on the rear legs to protect the fetlock from injuries. They are reinforced with rubber or thick leather heel patches. At a rodeo or other western event, you may notice stock and reining horses wearing skid boots. Also, any horse with a broken pastern angle should wear these boots while being worked because of the manner in which the back of the joint where the sesamoid bone is located drops to the ground and needs protection.

Galloping boots are a combination boot for tendon protection and support. They should provide protection to both the shin and ankle. A few manufacturers also make them for the hind legs.

Brush (brushing) boots are used during fox hunting and eventing. During construction, heavy-duty foam rubber is inserted to cushion the legs from concussion. These boots are lightweight and are intended for use under extreme competitive cross-country conditions.

Jumping boots or shin boots provide some tendon protection and support and are used in events such as the Hunter Division, Hunter Seat Equitation, and Jumping Division at shows. They may or may not have open fronts.

Weighted boots are a training aid for high-stepping, gaited horses such as Hackneys, Saddlebreds, and Morgans. These horses are schooled or ground driven while wearing these boots on the front feet. After the horse has been worked briefly during a training session, the lead-filled boots are removed and the horse's feet pop off the ground in a very showy style because his front feet are affected by the sudden "lightness." These boots are not used for protection, and the feet must have solid, strong hooves to maintain this activity. Special shoeing is also required.

Shipping boots are for trailering or vanning an equine. There are protective boots for the lower legs, as well as knee and hock coverings. Shipping boots are an excellent investment if you transport your horse frequently. The sturdy, well-padded boot with a bell-like covering over the pastern is excellent.

One economy shipping boot consists of quilted, padded squares with Velcro fasteners. Many horse owners and trainers use these in addition to bandages, especially for long trips. Most shipping boots, however, do not give the horse's legs any support.

Therapy boots are used to treat your horse's legs. There are simple types for sweating, and more complicated kinds

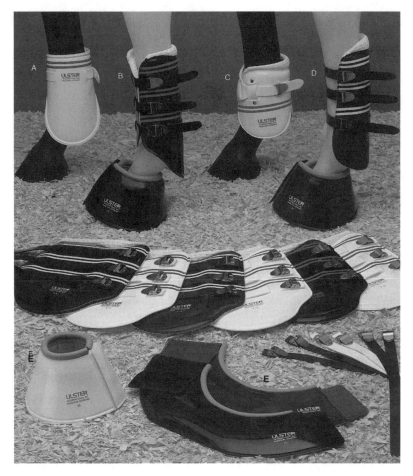

Performance horse boots made of man-made materials: a) half ankle; b) galloping or brush with tendon support; c) full ankle; d) open front brush boot; e) bell boot. The exteriors of these boots are vinyl and the interiors are shock absorbent Equilon. They are colorful and easy to care for, and have replaceable straps. _Courtesy of Ulster International, Inc._

for administering treatments, such as whirlpool baths. Others serve therapeutic purposes by providing temperature control, such as ice boots, and still others are used to medicate.

Sweat boots are used for sweating sore or swollen areas, such as fetlocks or hocks. These are usually of the ready-wrap type. Sweats are made of neoprene and foam rubber to induce sweating. Trainers often will use a sweat boot on a knee or hock for several hours instead of medication, or possibly for overnight relief. This type of boot is not used during exercising and is frequently applied along with standing wraps.

WORKING BOOTS FOR INTERFERING

Bell boots or overreach boots are probably the most common and least expensive boots used by trainers and owners. Whether or not your horse interferes, he will benefit from these cup-like pastern- and foot-covering boots. Bell boots, sometimes referred to as overreach boots, cover the pasterns, coronet bands, and heels. Hunters, polo ponies, and jumpers wear them to protect the coronet band, heels, and hoof walls from potential hard knocks and to prevent bruises and lacerations.

Ankle boots are used in all horse disciplines when the horse is overreaching (interfering). Some support is provided that will aid in reducing windpuffs. The sesamoid bones, which can fracture easily, are protected with a reinforced "heel." Another type of ankle boot is made especially to sweat swollen ankles.

CHOOSING THE RIGHT SIZE

Most vendors sell boots according to the weight and breed of your horse. Using only this information, however, may

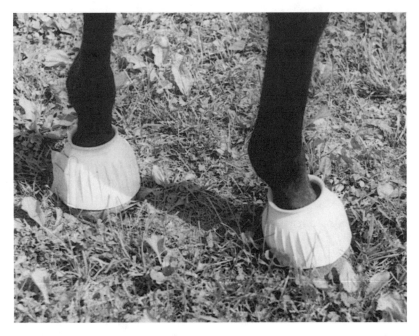

Popular rubber rib bell boots. These inexpensive boots give protection to the heels and coronet, as well as the front hoof, heel, and wall. They can be trimmed to shorten if necessary.

necessitate a return of merchandise if the fit is poor. Horses' legs, according to the manufacturers, come in small, medium, large and, occasionally, extra large. You may also find pony, cob, small horse, horse, and large horse sizes in your tack shop. To make fitting more complicated, a large horse may have a large leg with a short cannon bone, while a smaller breed may have a small leg circumference with a long cannon bone. Most boots are reasonably adjustable around the leg or pastern. If they fail to be high enough (two to three inches below the joints), however, or are too high, they do not fit.

When you are shopping, take your horse's leg and pastern measurements. Do not hesitate to order boots that are exactly the size you need. Proper fit is important not only to obtain the best results, but also to prevent injury. During a workout, a loose-fitting boot offers no support and will rub and irritate. If boots are too tight they can tear, and tight Velcro fasteners sometimes pop open. Even more important, a tight or loose boot could cause a bowed tendon or cording.

Methods of Measuring

Unless the tack vendor can travel to the horse barn to fit your horse, locate a flexible (cloth or soft plastic) tape and a pad and pencil. Since the lower rear legs of most horses are larger around and longer than the front legs, be sure to take rear-leg measurements if you are purchasing galloping, ankle, or skid boots and all four legs are to be covered.

Measure the lower leg by its circumference and length. Because the inside of the fetlock (ankle) is usually covered by the lower section of a boot (especially for splint protection or interference), include this area in both vertical and horizontal measurements.

Hold the tape vertically on one of the legs to be fitted and write down the following measurements:

1. Start from below the knee or hock and run the tape down the front to where the ankle just flexes.

2. Then measure inside the leg, from the knee to below the fetlock joint.

3. Next, make note of the leg's circumference by measuring horizontally around the leg just below the knee or hock.

4. Finally, measure around the leg just above the fetlock (ankle), but not including the joint, and also around the ankle including the joint at its widest point (this measurement may or may not be needed).

With these measurements, you should be well prepared when approaching a tack shop in search of lower-leg protection for your horse. To double-check a purchase, make sure that the buckles or closures have ample room for fastening, especially if your horse still has some developing to do. Before going to the cashier, buckle the boots using a hole about in the center and measure the circumference with your cloth tape.

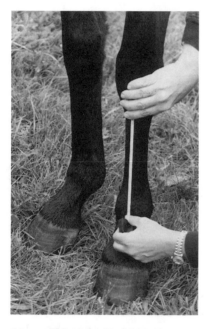

Measure the length of the cannon bone for height. Hold the end of the tape immediately below the knee (or hock) joint and at the flexion point of the ankle. Measure and fit carefully so that the boots do not rub while the horse is moving.

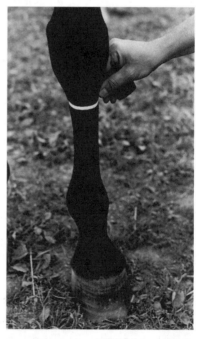

Measure the circumference of the upper cannon bone area.

Measuring for Boots that Protect Pasterns and Heels

For a pair of bell boots, measure the circumference of the front feet, which encompasses the pastern area and the hoof. Wrap the tape above the coronet band for the circumference. For height, measure from the pastern to the tip of the toe at the front and from the coronet band down the back of the heel. If rubber cup bell boots are too long, but the next size smaller is too tight or does not cover the front sufficiently, you can trim them. The important areas to cover are the coronary band and the heels.

Foot sizes vary. Knowing your horse's shoe size will be an aid in buying boots for the feet. This information may be obtained from your blacksmith.

BOOT CARE

You must keep leather and fabric boots, as well as bell boots, clean and in good condition if they are to function properly. Dirt wears boots quickly and irritates legs. A brushing or damp wipe plus application of conditioner will usually suffice. After your horse has a workout in mud, you will need to apply a bit more energy. Five or ten minutes of cleaning with a mild saddle or oil soap immediately after working will preserve leather boots. Saddle conditioner or oil will keep them fresh and flexible. Apply after the leather is clean and dry.

Plastic or vinyl boots may be rinsed or wiped with a damp cloth. Take care not to soak the padded lining. Do not be deceived by the notion that soaking the boots will get them cleaner—you may damage them. If soap is necessary for badly soiled vinyl, sponge it off thoroughly.

Some manufacturers claim that their poly and vinyl products can be cleaned in a clothes washer with the rest of the horse's laundry. However, they must be air dried; never put them into a dryer! Check the care instruction labels.

Bell boots, especially, become grimy. Rubber or vinyl bell boots should be swished around in a pail of soapy water, then rinsed. When they are stained with oiled arena footing, a good brushing will clean them, but the stains often remain. The inside of the boots should be spotless—no grit to rub against your horse's coronary band.

Buying good boots to keep all four of your horse's legs protected is an expensive investment, but to what lengths will a good horse owner go to protect his horse? Boots can also be an attractive accessory, but keep in mind their purpose when you decide to buy them.

The decision about any special boots for your horse should be left up to an experienced horseman, or preferably, a trainer.

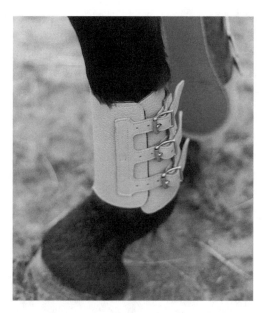

When boots are installed, the buckles should utilize the holes nearest the center of the tab. Often the bottom buckle fastens larger. Use the same holes on botyh boots so the support matches on both legs.

CHAPTER 6
Leg Injuries That
Require Bandaging

This chapter is intended as an aid in caring for and identifying a few common leg problems suffered by horses. A leg injury may occur at almost anytime—during a workout, while the horse is being hauled, or when pastured with other horses. The causes for some of these leg traumas are provided so you can employ preventive maintenance. However, it is important that you learn to detect *any* lameness in your horse. Ask your veterinarian to explain what he sees when your horse is moving that indicates soreness.

Please understand that this text is not intended to be used for diagnosis or "do-it-yourself" treatments (that is the veterinarian's job), but it has been prepared to enhance your understanding of trauma and enable you to follow your veterinarian's instructions.

Dressings are difficult to maintain on a horse, which is why a bandage is usually used for only a few days. A bandage dressing is essential where a wound or abscess is draining, or to keep medication in place. Use a dressing to protect a deep injury or surgical opening, muffle a bleeding wound, and/or keep out foreign matter.

The concerned horse owner will discover that caring for her sick or injured animal is similar to nursing a sick child back to health. Your horse is dependent on you for his recovery. The information contained herein is intended to aid you in following your veterinarian's instructions.

TYPES OF LEG AILMENTS

Your horse must always be kept clean and dry, especially during warm, humid weather. If dirt and mud are permitted to accumulate on his legs for long periods of time, skin eruptions will develop.

Fungus, Bacteria, Scabs, Scratches

Fungus infestations become a problem for horse owners during damp, humid weather, especially during the spring. A horse's legs can develop small sores or rashes caused by yeast or fungus, which then become infected with bacteria. These scabs and sores will spread if not treated immediately.

Scratches are rash-like sores, fungal eruptions on the skin of your horse's legs resulting in scales or scabs. Bacteria set up colonies within the pus-filled sores underneath these scabs. This irritation may both itch and be painful. It is difficult to cure, but the fungus can be controlled. The sores usually start in the soft skin above the heels and under the fetlocks. Sometimes this infestation is severe, called "mud fever." The horse may have a low-grade temperature.

Summer itch, a warm weather rash, which may or may not begin on the legs, consists of small itching sores which spread when the horse attempts to scratch the discomfort. It will eventually cover a large portion or all of his body.

Ringworm, another common problem, is contagious to other livestock and to humans.

Dry skin patches with hair loss are usually caused by yeast.

A good iodine shampoo on your horse's legs and body, even (carefully) on his face, during the first warm days of spring should curtail the onset of these infestations. If you do

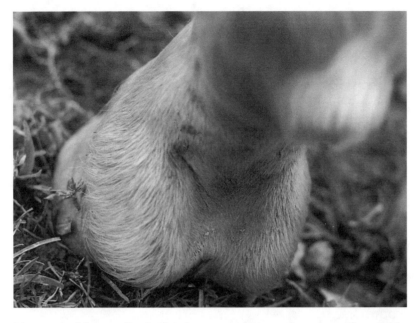

The onset of fungus. To check it from spreading, wash pasterns thoroughly with iodine shampoo and apply antiseptic ointment. Within three days all evidence of the condition should disappear.

not have iodine shampoo, following his bath, drench him in a Betadine Solution, then scrape him down and dry him.

Should rash-like scabs already be in evidence and spreading, after shampooing, scrape off all the scabs, then saturate these areas with full-strength Betadine Solution. The scabs remove easily after being softened by bathing. An antiseptic ointment may be applied on the sores while your horse is drying. With the scabs off, the antiseptic and medication have access to the sores. If a few scabs are present a day or so later, spot treat a second time.

If the back of the horse's pasterns and legs have become nearly raw from irritation, after a thorough cleansing and removal of scabs off all four feet and legs, cover the raw areas generously with furacin or nitrofurazone ointment and cover with plastic or wax paper (one layer only) to keep the salve moist and in place. Apply stall wraps over the plastic or paper for a secure bandage. Of course, your horse must be kept in his stall while bandaged during the next twelve hours. The following day leave the legs uncovered so air can get at the raw sores and aid in healing.

An antifungal product may be applied at this time. Follow the instructions on the label. An anti-fungal solution or iodine solution should be re-applied once or twice within the following week(s) until all signs of the sores disappear. Antifungal solutions are available in spray containers.

Treating Minor Injuries

Accidents will occur during turnout when there is activity among a herd. Therefore, attempt to avoid as many hurts and ouches as possible by providing a safe environment for your horse.

To treat minor cuts and scratches, or insect bites, merely rinse the wound with cool, slow-running water from the hose. The flowing water flushes out dirt or debris and the coolness relieves discomfort.

If the horse has taken a little skin off his leg, daily care of this or a minor cut may consist of no more than rinsing with running water and applying diluted Betadine Solution or antibacterial salve. If heat or swelling is noted, the horse's legs are put into standing wraps, and he is placed in a quiet stall.

Within twenty-four hours, a minor injury begins to dry, at which time, after rinsing to remove any dirt, apply an antiseptic ointment or a furazone. When an injury occurs on the top of a knee or ankle, the scab must be kept soft and elastic to enable the joint to function. Fura ointment combined with bandaging should keep the wound soft while healing. These wounds must heal from the inside, and any thick scab must be removed.

Ask your veterinarian for instructions when serious injuries occur. They require immediate medical attention. For example, if a puncture wound is hot and filled with pus, DO NOT APPLY ANY WATER unless the veterinarian instructs you. This also applies where there is a deep wound or one that covers a large area. Keep your horse quiet, preferably in a stall, until examined and treated.

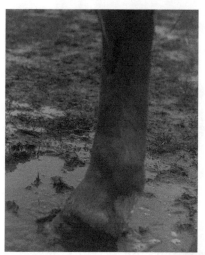

A minor wound such as this can be hosed to clean out dirt and reduce pain. Fura ointment should be applied to the scrapes to keep the area soft and keep bacteria from developing.

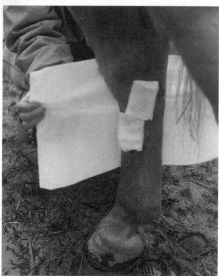

The following day the leg had swollen. Standing wraps were necessary because of the swelling. The leg was rinsed, Fura ointment reapplied, and gauze patches placed over the raw areas.

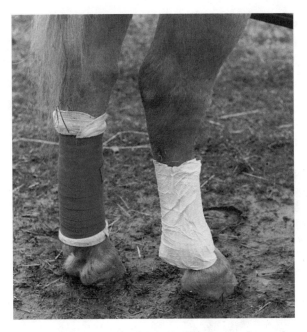

Paper towel or a cotton sheet must be wrapped over the gauze to keep it in place and prevent the quilt from sticking. Always remember to wrap *all* four legs.

Standing wraps will be necessary for a badly skinned, swollen leg. First, hose the leg with cold water long enough to cool and cleanse it, then treat the raw areas with an antibacterial ointment such as Fura. Apply gauze squares to protect the injury from irritation. Never wrap rolled gauze around a horse's leg because it will bind. You can use a cotton sheet made for leg wrapping or a plain paper towel to further protect the skinned areas and keep the medication off the quilts. The sheet or paper permits some air to enter. Never use plastic on this type of injury because the wound must breathe. The cotton or paper towel allows some air to reach the wound, aiding the healing process. Then apply quilt wraps over the sheet. Put the other three legs into standing wraps as well.

A dressing or light bandage may be a waste of time on an injury that your horse can easily reach with his mouth. If there is pain and/or itching, your horse will probably attempt to lick the wound and will eventually pull the dressing off. A neck cradle can be used for a few hours to keep him from disturbing the bandage, but excessive use of this device is unwarranted.

When a horse refuses to leave a dressing alone, determine if discomfort may be the reason. The bandage may be too tight, or the wound may be infected or very painful. Investigate and treat the cause to enhance proper healing and comfort of your horse.

Articular Windpuffs

Windpuffs are associated with young horses under heavy training programs and overworked older horses. A windpuff is a soft lump on the fetlock; an inflamation on the joint capsule. No heat is evident on or around this puffy spot, and there rarely is lameness. The blemish is permanent.

The horse is not worked and his legs should be kept in standing wraps until your veterinarian prescribes hand walking or quiet turnout. Sweat boots may be used if your veterinarian recommends them.

LEG PROBLEMS OF OLDER HORSES

Horses that have been worked hard all their lives will have old injuries, and arthritis will flare up now and then. These aches and pains must be dealt with on an ongoing basis by your veterinarian.

Any degenerative joint problem is not only painful, but can become disabling. A good hosing with cold water to cool and a gentle liniment rub will give some comfort to your horse.

When your older horse begins to walk stiffly out of his stall after standing in it for several hours, he is developing joint problems. He should be walked out slowly. After he has been turned out half an hour or so, the kinks will gradually disappear. Stall wraps each night while your older horse is being worked will make him more comfortable.

If your working horse begins to develop severe joint prob-

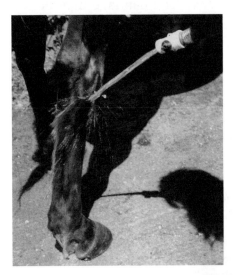

Hosing sore joints with cold water relieves much of the discomfort and reduces heating in the leg.

After a hard workout, hose the legs down and apply full stength liniment. This provides cold and warm therapy combined with massage.

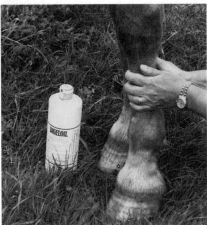

lems, he frequently will exhibit soreness and sometimes heat may be felt in the area of irritation. At this point, night wraps will be necessary along with prescribed medications.

Care of Sore Joints

Performance horses suffer much too often with "bad hocks." Jumpers and field hunters, in particular, develop osteoarthritis in one or both hocks. Each hock consists of four joints, two upper and two lower. If your horse is in the midst of a show season when he gets sore, injections in the hock may keep him going pain-free until the season ends.

Sweating a joint is an old timer's treatment, and a good one because no chemicals or medicinals need be used. Sweating an ankle, a front knee, or a hock should not present any behavior problems, even though your horse is restricted. Your horse may become riled if he feels trapped. His first sweating experience should be done in an open area. (The treatment is usually done in a stall or while the horse is standing in a quiet aisle.) Be prepared for an argument or a blowup when he discovers that his leg will not bend normally. Choose a place where there are no walls, gates, or solid objects for him to kick or bump into, and tie him to a strong post. If no post is available, get someone to assist.

Go slowly. Apply one sweat boot at a time. Take care that the boots do not slip down. A horse may either try to bolt forward, buck, or walk backwards while kicking to get rid of what is holding his legs. Do not encourage him to do any walking while the boots are in place, because this serves to remind him that he is restricted. A hay bag tied within easy reach should keep him busy.

Sweating takes two to three hours, or possibly longer. Follow your veterinarian's instructions as to how long and on what schedule. Your horse must be observed or monitored during the treatment. Sweating is more effective when the horse is already warm from exercise. If the weather is cold and he is being rested, a sweating solution may be applied to the area of the leg to be treated and then rinsed off later. The boots need to be thoroughly washed after each use.

Chronic Lameness Due to Back Pain

Never discount having your vet thoroughly examine your horse's back when there is lameness, especially when it is chronic. Performing mares will occasionally display lameness and a sore back in the spring. They may have stiffness along one side, including the neck, and may limp slightly and prefer their forehand. Mares may be irritable and argue about being mounted. These symptoms suggest that the ovaries should be examined. Night wraps on all four legs will make the mare more comfortable until the pain subsides. Acupuncture treatments, along with hot compresses over the sore area and liniment massages, seem to work wonders on most of these mares.

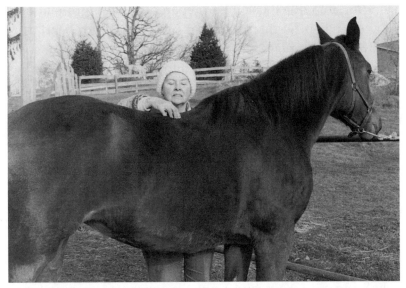

Use your fingertips to locate sensitive areas in the back after riding.

METHODS OF THERAPY

Liniments and braces followed with a massage and standing wraps is a daily routine in a working barn. Absorbine liniment or Bigeloil can be massaged on full strength—after a bath or good hosing—when a strong solution is required, or it may be diluted and sponged on as a body wash and brace. Full-strength applications of liniment or rubbing alcohol are used for muscle spasms and soreness. They are gently but firmly rubbed on the horse's wet legs or back. In this instance, the legs must be thoroughly dried before standing wraps are applied.

For a body and leg wash or brace, follow the instructions on the label, but generally the solution consists of one to two ounces of liniment to two quarts of warm water, per horse. Apply while warm. During very cold weather, body rinsing should be avoided unless the barn is heated and draft-free. If your horse is to be stabled, he should be dry when placed in his stall for the night.

COLD THERAPY

Immersion or Hosing

Cold treatments (hypothermia) are used during the first twenty-four to forty-eight hours following trauma, and are often used for leg injuries which exhibit swelling and/or "hot spots," as well as for burns and minor scrapes and cuts. Cold therapy is of little value after forty-eight hours except when alternating hot and cold, such as when treating a sprain or minor fracture. Cold therapy may consist of cold water hosing or immersion, ice packs, cold wet quilts, or an application of cooling gel on the horse's legs and feet. It is probably one of the most frequent types of first aid therapy.

Hosing with cold water after a schooling session is suggested to relieve aches and prevent edema or tissue swelling.

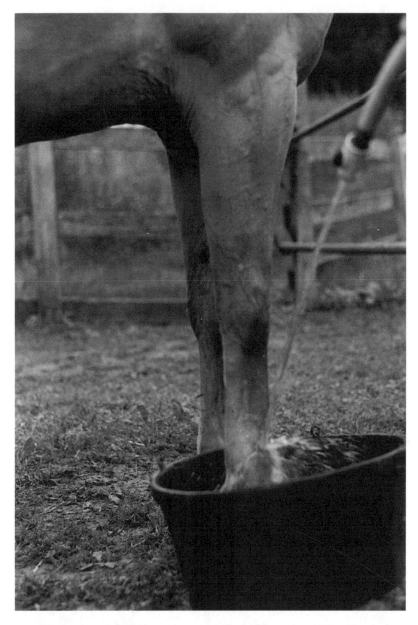

A cold water soak plus hosing to cool the ankle and pastern. The foot is placed in an empty tub, then water is hosed over the troubled area for about five minutes. Let the cold water cover the fetlock for a few additional minutes of soaking.

Should a warm limb or a hot spot be found, at least ten to fifteen minutes of cold water hosing or soaking should immediately be directed upon that site.

After about fifteen minutes of cold therapy, the horse's legs are wrapped and he is rested, preferably in a stall to limit activity and further trauma and/or swelling. If another cold treatment is necessary, wait at least one hour. When your veterinarian orders half-hour to forty-five-minute daily cold water therapy sessions, they should be scheduled throughout the day to provide an ongoing, regular cooling of the afflicted tissues. When extended cooling of the tissue is required, cold, wet wraps or ice may be utilized, as well as a cold gel. (See the section on poultices and gels.)

The hoof walls need drying time. Treatment which includes the immersion of a foot in water should not exceed forty-five minutes within a twenty-four hour period. If you notice the white line separating from the hoof wall (lumen), discontinue immersion and have your horse's feet trimmed and checked for abscess or a condition known as "seedy toe."

Swimming and wading pools provide excellent therapeutic and rehabilitative exercise for leg problems.

Ice Packs

Considerable trauma and swelling requires that the tissue be cooled with crushed ice or small frozen (two-to-three-inch square) ice packets. Ice boots that provide approximately two hours of cold treatment are also available.

Packets or ice cells with quick-freeze solution can be tucked into Professional Medicine Boots or inside polo wraps for cold treatments. These small packets can be kept in a freezer so they are readily available. The ice is contained, so it keeps the limb dry. Homemade ice packets made with loose, crushed ice contained in small plastic bags can also be used

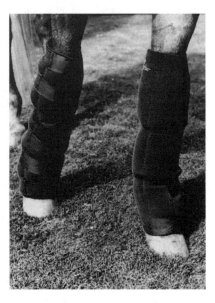

One type of ice boot. The nine pocket ice boot has pockets which hold packets of ice. The portable packs can be kept in a freezer until needed.
Courtesy of Professional's Choice Sports Medicine Products, Inc.

under quilts. The homemade packet must be flexible so it can form around the horse's leg or pastern.

Cold, Wet Quilts

Another form of cool therapy is the use of wet quilts with overnight or twelve-hour standing wraps. This kind of therapy can also be applied after a hard workout and on old, healed injuries that become troublesome occasionally. Medium-weight quilts are saturated with water, rolled, and placed in the freezer for a couple of hours before applying to your horse's leg(s). The frozen condition does not last long, but has a quick cooling effect.

Wet Treatment of an Open Wound

Another caution: Moist therapy, such as wet standing wraps, whirlpool, or soaking cannot be used where there is an open wound. A "dry cold" utilizing ice may be applied to reduce any swelling. Wet treatments, such as moist wraps or whirlpool, are avoided because they will

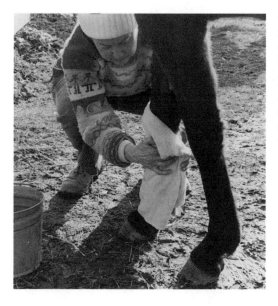

To focus warmth where needed, apply a warm compress around the horse's leg.
A heavy bath towel which holds warm water well and is easy to wash afterward makes an excellent warm compress.

admit bacteria into the wound and cause infection.

Heat Therapy

Applying heat to an injury begins twenty-four to forty-eight hours after a trauma has been sustained. Warm applications stimulate the limb's circulation. Heat therapy is not applied where infection is present. Its use may spread the infection. Only under your vet's supervision should warm water treatment in conjunction with medication be utilized to draw out pus.

Mild exercise or massage usually follows the application of heat. For injuries demanding total rest, a turbulator device or whirlpool warm water bath may provide passive massage.

The conductive heat consists of hot water at 120 degrees Fahrenheit. You can test the temperature by submerging your elbow into the water. During cold weather, the warm bath water or soak must be re-warmed before the end of the treatment. Take care not to pour hot water directly onto the injured limb.

Wet towels (compresses) are folded and applied by hand after squeezing out the excess heated water.

Combining Heat and Cold Therapy

Alternating cold with heat is often used on long healing injuries. Applying cold water or ice, then spreading on a warming poultice, is one method. Another is to follow a warm water soak or compress treatment with an ice gel or ice boot.

These treatments should be used only on the advice of a veterinarian.

POULTICES AND GELS

A veterinarian may suggest that you apply poultices (prepared pastes or salves) or ice gels to therapeutically assist in healing as well as to reduce pain. They provide hours of relief when used properly. After applying the compound, wrap the horse's leg in one layer of either Kraft paper or plastic wrap, covered by a quilt wrap, then finish with standing bandages. Poultices and ice gels are intended to prolong a warm or cold treatment, respectively, when properly applied and left on for several hours.

After exertion, poultices or gels may also be left on your horse's legs overnight with standing wraps. The following morning the wraps are removed and the poultice is washed away with running water.

Black drawing salves act as poultices on abscesses and puncture wounds. They are often used following a soaking or an application of hot compresses, and are applied with a dry compress covered by a plastic wrap under a standing bandage. When applied on your horse's feet, poultice boots

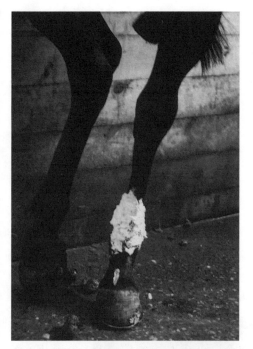

A poultice may be either
cold or warming.
Here a poultice has
been applied
to the lower leg.

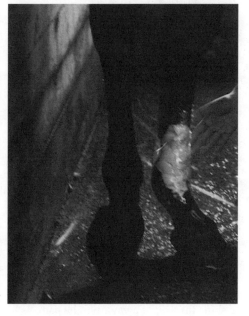

Plastic wrap is applied
over the poultice
to keep it moist
and to avoid soiling
the wrap.

A quilt is applied over the plastic
wrap and the legs
are put in
standing bandages.

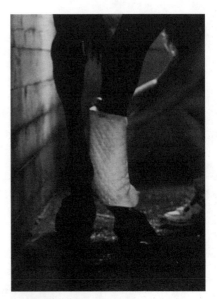

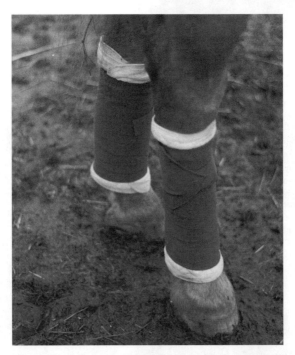

Remember to wrap both legs: the injured one to minimize swelling, and the opposite leg for support when the horse shifts his weight away from the pain.

or wraps must be used to keep the wound clean and the medication in place.

COMPLETE STALL REST

Confinement ideally takes place in a twelve-by-eighteen-foot foaling stall. This provides space for use of therapeutic equipment which otherwise must be placed in the aisle. Some serious leg injuries dictate a more restrictive confinement, such as tying the horse in a straight stall or in a large stall with a corner-tie or cross-tie. Always tie the horse with the rope(s) head high. Water and hay should be hung high and well within reach so it is not necessary for him to move around very much to satisfy thirst or hunger.

Your horse's legs should always be wrapped when he is confined to his stall for any length of time. The lower legs tend to swell from standing without exercise—that is probably why the term "standing wraps" originated.

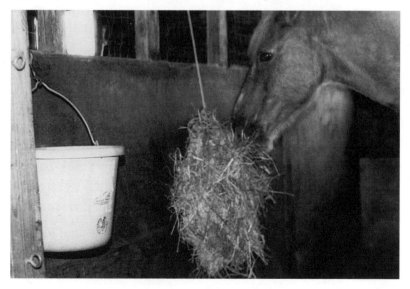

A quiet stall is necessary for recovery. Extra hay will keep the horse content until the sore leg heels enough for walking or turnout. Grain rations are usually either eliminated or cut back.

CONCLUSION

Throughout this book, protecting the legs of young horses in training, horses being "brought back," and performance or working horses has been stressed by recommending the use of bandages or boots. This is an individual decision. However, you should not approach this issue with the rationalization that "I don't have enough time to wrap." A young horse is like a time capsule—every experience, each large or small trauma, is remembered and comes home with age.

Proper horse care is time consuming, but rewarding. When a horse owner is consistent each day, maintaining a regular schedule and using preventive maintenance, his horse is not only content, but has fewer problems later on. The ideal situation is, of course, to start proper leg care from the moment the foal hits the ground and continue care and maintenance throughout his entire lifetime. Upon reaching the grand old age of, say, twenty-eight, barring accidents, your horse's legs and feet should be in as good a condition as they were when he was ten.

There are few things more beautiful than a healthy, well mannered horse or pony. Man takes care of 'em and God blesses 'em.

GLOSSARY

ABSCESS — a concentration of pus beneath the skin, sometimes quite deep, caused by an infection. An abscess may be caused by the intrusion of an embedded foreign object or a hard knock that produces a deep bruise.

ARTICULAR — relating to a joint.

BABY SITTER — A compatible, older horse that is a young horse's companion and oftentimes teacher.

BACK OR BACKING A HORSE — to gradually apply weight on a horse's back to acquaint him with how to balance the weight and ready him for being ridden.

BIOTIN — an amino acid which aids a horse's healthy growth of hair and hooves when ingested regularly. Biotin, combined with other nutrients, can be supplemented in the horse's diet.

BLOWUP — when a horse blows up, it is because he becomes overly frightened and excited. He will be difficult to hold, his legs kicking in all directions. They often rear and/or buck vigorously, and will attempt to escape their handler by yanking on the lead line. If loose, they will sometimes bolt and run away.

BOWED TENDON — a trauma causing the thickening (bulging) of the superficial flexor tendon, usually between the knee or hock and the fetlock.

BREAK — to teach discipline, such as halter breaking, for riding or driving.

BREAKOVER — the manner in which the horse applies weight on his foot as he travels forward, e.g. heel, center, and over the toe. The breakover point is how the toe breaks into the ground at completion of stride. A good breakover is centered at the toe.

CHESTNUTS — dry leathery outgrowths on the inside of each leg.

CHRONIC — a persistent or recurring malady.

COB — indicates the size of a horse. A small horse between 14 to 15 hand high, excepting the "Welsh Cob," which is a breed.

COGGINS TEST — blood test for the presence of antibodies against the often fatal equine infectious anemia (EIA) virus.

COLD SHOE — a horseshoe prepared and shaped without heating.

COLLAGEN FIBERS — connective tissue (removed from a deceased animal) which is an insoluble protein fiber used to patch living tissue.

COLLECT — to impulse the hindquarters so that the horse brings his rear legs slightly under, shortening his strides. In so doing, the horse's back lifts and his neck flexes.

COMPOUND FRACTURE — a complete break of a bone.

COOL OUT OR COOL DOWN — to walk a heated (possibly sweating) horse to relax him emotionally and lower his body temperature after working or when he has been overly excited. This may take ten to thirty minutes (no cold water is given to drink) and the horse is usually covered to avoid cold air chills. This procedure aids the body to slowly throw off toxicity build-up that can cause muscle tie up.

CORDING — swelling of a dleg due to the circulation being shut off. Soft tissue could atrophy if the offensive binding is not removed quickly enough. Often when a leg cords up it swells to twice its normal size.

CORONARY BAND OR CUSHION — the rise above the coronet.

CORONET BAND — is the area from which the hoof wall grows. It is soft and sensitive, e.g. should the coronet be damaged, the hoof will not grow normally from that point until the area heals.

CURB —thickening of the tendon or ligament, with the enlargement at the back of the hock.

DMSO — Dimethyl sulfoxide, a naturally occurring chemical that is able to pass through the skin. It contains anti-inflammatory, antibacterial and analgesic properties.

DRESSAGE — a disciplined technique for both horse and rider where the horse and rider become as "one," working together. After undergoing extensive training there are a series of tests where the horse's performance is scrupulously judged.

EDEMA — an accumulation of water in the cellular tissue creating a swollen condition.

ERGOT — a dry pointed growth located at the rear of each fetlock. If they become too long, they can be trimmed with scissors.

FETLOCK JOINT — sometimes referred to as the ankle, joins the pastern and cannon bone (at the second phalanx or short pastern bone).

FOALING STALL — a double- or triple-sized box stall, approximately 12 by 18 or 24 feet. The additional space is used during foaling for equipment and ample space for a medical team to work if need be. The foal requires the added space also.

FOOTPRINTING — occurs as a parallel rear foot comes forward and steps into or near the footprint of the forefoot.

FOREHAND — the front of the horse, from the withers through the shoulders and forelegs. When it is said the horse is on his forehand, he is heaviest on his front feet while moving forward.

GREEN HORSE — one that is not fully trained and young.

GREEN OSSELET — an inflammation at the fetlock joint or damage to the articular cartilage at the front of the cannon and/or pastern bones. If there is an excess of synovial fluid it leads to a condition referred to as an articular windpuff.

HOT SPOT — a term used to describe an area on a foot or leg found to be much warmer than neighboring areas or the opposite limb.

IMPLANT — to surgically embed or insert into a living site where it becomes a biological part of and grows with the living tissue.

LONG REIN — ground drive; a term used in horse training. It means to work a horse from the ground using two long reins and following behind or to the side.

LONGEING — moving a horse around, circling the trainer, on a longe line approximately twenty-five feet in length. A whip is held to encourage either forward movement, engagement of quarters, and to slow or to halt. The enclosed working area is square or round, fifty to sixty feet across, with secure footing. Longeing is a teaching method during which your horse learns both manners and confidence while he builds muscle. He also learns balance and cadence while being prepared for riding. A thorough knowledge of how to longe should be acquired before anyone should undertake the practice because much training can be "undone" by inexperienced hands.

METHIONINE — an amino acid which promotes healthy hoof growth and can be fed as a supplement.

OILED — dosing a horse with mineral oil to clean out the digestive tract and bowels.

OVERHEATED HORSE — a horse that has run or been worked too long and too hard. Overheating occurs more often in summer heat with high humidity. Feeling the center of your horse's chest and watching the rise and fall of his breath rate at the loin are good sensing points for a hot horse. The horse may or may not be sweating profusely, pulse rate is rapid and his body will feel very hot to the palm of handler's hand. The overexerted, hot horse will stand with its feet spread for support and its head hanging when not cooled immediately. If not attended, he will go down and expire.

PACER — a racing horse that trots laterally. He moves both legs on each side instead of diagonally the way a trotting horse does.

PADDOCK — an individual turnout area which may be half an acre or larger enclosed with proper fencing, with a supply of drinking water. The large breeds, such as Thoroughbreds or European Warmbloods, require larger paddocks because they need room to romp without hitting their legs or feet against solid objects.

PASTERN — the leg segment between the fetlock joint and the coronet band. Respectively, the first phalanx or long pastern bone, and the second phalanx or short pastern bone.

PHENYLBUTAZONE — (bute) a drug which alleviates pain and is an anti-inflammatory agent.

PLAITING ACTION — an extreme interference where the forelegs cross in transit.

PONYING — a horse led by a rider on horseback.

PROUD FLESH — an excessive growth of granular tissue (scar).

RINGWORM — a skin disease caused by fungus. It is contagious. Circular, rash-like patches leave skin bare and slightly swollen.

SHIPPING FEVER — a bacterial and metabolic illness that arises when adrenal glands are overworked; caused by prolonged physical stress.

SIDEBONE — hard, bony lump at the back side of the horse's coronet.

SPLINT BONES — slender bones situated on either side of the cannon bone.

STIFLE JOINT — joint junctioning the tibia and patella. This joint is positioned to flex the horse's rear knee.

STOCKING-UP — swelling of legs usually due to lack of exercise such as during stall confinement.

STRINGHALT — a nervous disorder which causes the horse to snatch up a hind leg briefly while walking or trotting; thought to be inherited.

SUBLUXATION — a misalignment of a joint or joints, or vertebrae.

SYNOVIAL FLUID — nature's joint oil.

TELLINGTON TOUCH — a method of acutouch done to diagnose and treat. Discovered by Linda Tellington Jones, a horse trainer, and used by professional practitioners.

THROMBOSIS — blood clotting within a vein or artery of living tissue.

TYING-UP — azoturia; an extremely painful, severe cramping in the quarters or possibly in the shoulder muscle masses. The horse's urine may discolor.

RECOMMENDED READING

ADAMS' LAMENESS IN HORSES, (Ed.) Stashak, T.S., 4th Ed. Lea & Febinger, Philadelphia, 1987.

BEGINNER'S GUIDE TO HORSES: BUYING, EQUIPPING, AND STA-BLING, Melcher, Carol R., A.S. Barnes & Co., Inc., Cranbury, NJ, 1974.

THE BODY LANGUAGE OF HORSES, Ainslie, Tom, and Ledbetter, Bonnie, Wm. Morrow and Co., Inc., NY, 1980.

CENTERED RIDING, Swift, Sally, St. Martin's/Marek, NY, 1985.

EQUINE HOOF CARE, Trapani, J., Arco Publishing, Inc., NY, 1983.

THE LAME HORSE, Rooney, James R., Wilshire Book Co., N. Holly-wood, CA, 1984.

THERE ARE NO PROBLEM HORSES, ONLY PROBLEM RIDERS, Twelveponies, Mary, Houghton Mifflin Co., Boston, 1982.

RIDING LOGIC, Museler, Wilhelm, 4th Ed., Arco Publishing, Inc., NY, . 1973.

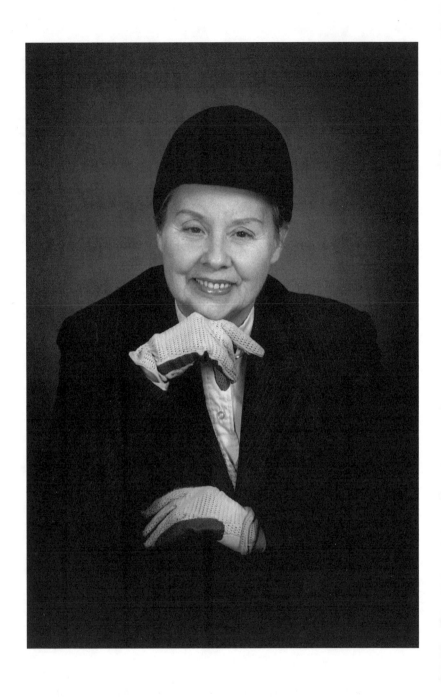

About the Author

Born in Michigan, Sue Allen discovered the quiet joy of horses long before attending school. Her father kept a family horse and a neighbor raised Thoroughbreds. She fondly recalls climbing through the fence and catching a horse in the pasture to sneak a bareback joy ride.

While taking classes at NYU, she spent her leisure time at jumping classes or riding a hack in Central Park. Soon she added equestrian arts and horse training techniques to her journalism studies. After studying in New York, Sue made teaching and writing an important part of her life. For ten years she was a member of the health sciences staff at Columbia University in New York. On the weekends and evenings she taught hunt seat in Westchester and Southern Dutchess county show barns, and eventually started a small riding school of her own. She trained and exhibited her own horses from 1986 to 1993.

A back injury unhappily put a stop to a heavy showing schedule, and eventually the school had to be set aside. Sue turned her attention back to writing and, seeing a need for riding students to learn how to protect the valuable legs on their mounts, continued giving leg care clinics at riding schools. Her assessment of the need for more information on the subject led to the writing of this book. Other books on foot and leg care are planned for the future.

Sue Allen's articles and photography have been published in *Horseman, Horseplay, The Chronicle of the Horse, Horse and*

Horseman , *Poughkeepsie Journal, Southern Duchess News, Hudson Valley Magazine,* and others .

Anyone who loves horses becomes wonderfully addicted to them, Sue claims. Working around horses remains a major part of her life. Sue takes her Anglo-Arab mare with her across the country, and she occasionally takes on the training of a young horse or a serious rider.

Your Comments are Invited

If you found *How to Use Leg Wraps, Bandage,s and Boots,* especially helpful, or if you have other comments on this title, we would like to hear from you. Just write:

Editorial Office
Alpine Publications
225 S. Madison Ave.
Loveland, CO 80537

We'll send you a FREE coupon for your efforts!

For a Free Catalog of Alpine Titles

or information on any other Alpine books, please write or call our Customer Service Department at P. O. Box 7027, Loveland, CO 80537, or toll free 1-800-777-7257.

Additional Titles of Interest:

Coloring Atlas of
HORSE ANATOMY
Robert A. Kainer, DVM
and Thomas O. McCracken, M.S.

Influencing Horse Behavior
Dr. Jim McCall

Horse Training Basics
Deborah M. Britt